China's Sports Medicine

Medicine and Sport Science

Founder and Editor from 1969 to 1984
E. Jokl, Lexington, Ky.

Vol. 28

Series Editors
M. Hebbelinck, Brussels
R.J. Shephard, Toronto, Ont.

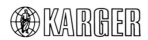

Basel · München · Paris · London · New York · New Delhi · Singapore · Tokyo · Sydney

China's Sports Medicine

Volume Editors
Qu Mianyu, Beijing
Yu Changlong, Beijing

46 figures and 51 tables, 1988

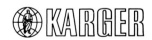 KARGER

Basel · München · Paris · London · New York · New Delhi · Singapore · Tokyo · Sydney

Medicine and Sport Science

Published on behalf of the Research Committee of the International Council of Sport Sciences and Physical Education

Library of Congress Cataloging-in-Publication Data
China's sports medicine.
(Medicine and sport science; vol. 28)
Includes bibliographies and index.
1. Sports medicine – China. I. Qu Mianyu. II. Yu Changlong. III. Series.
[DNLM: 1. Sports Medicine – China. WI ME649Q v. 28/QT 260 C5385]
RC1210.C54 1988 617'.1027'0951 88-13173
ISBN 3-8055-4806-0

Drug Dosage
The authors and the publisher have exerted every effort to ensure that drug selection and dosage set forth in this text are in accord with current recommendations and practice at the time of publication. However, in view of ongoing research, changes in government regulations, and the constant flow of information relating to drug therapy and drug reactions, the reader is urged to check the package insert for each drug for any change in indications and dosage and for added warnings and precautions. This is particularly important when the recommended agent is a new and/or infrequently employed drug.

Contents

Preface VII

Qu Mianyu (Beijing): Sports Medicine in China 1
Qu Mianyu; Yu Changlong (Beijing): Clinical and Pathological
   Studies on Enthesiopathy of Athletes 7
Qu Mianyu (Beijing): The Pathophysiology and Principles of Rehabil-
   itation after Cartilage Injury 19
Gao Yunqiu; Pu Junzong; Zhang Baohui (Beijing): Long-Term
   Follow-Up Study of Abnormal Electrocardiograms in Athletes . 34
Pu Junzong (Beijing): Exercise-Induced Urinary Abnormalities in
   Athletes 43
Duan Weijiang; Qiao Juxiang (Beijing): Anaerobic Performance of
   Chinese Untrained and Trained 11- to 18-Year-Old Boys and
   Girls 52
Fan Zhenhua; Chen Xiner; Tu Danyun (Shanghai): Functional Train-
   ing after Reconstruction of the Thumb through Free Transplanta-
   tion of the Second Toe 61
Xu Shengwen; Fan Zhenhua (Shanghai): Physiological Studies of Tai
   Ji Quan in China 70
Zhou Shifang; Cao Guohua; Jing Yu; Li Jianan (Nanjing): Effects of
   Aerobic Training and Qigong on the Prostacyclin-Thromboxane
   A_2 Balance of Patients with Coronary Heart Disease 81
Lu Dinghou; Duan Changping; Zhang Jianguo; Fan Jingyu; Tang
   Xiaojing (Beijing): Effect of Acupuncture on Ultrastructural
   Alteration in Skeletal Muscle after Strenuous Exercise 90
Ji Di Chen (Beijing): Some Sports Nutrition Researches in China . . 94

Subject Index 115

Preface

Although China has a long history of therapeutic exercise, practice in treatment, prevention of diseases and prolonging people's life, all of which plays an important role in sports medicine, sports medicine as a comprehensive scientific modern science has only a short history of about 30 years in China.

The purpose of this book 'China's Sports Medicine' is to give a brief introduction of the past and present situation concerning clinical and research work in sports medicine in China. Eleven representative papers are included. I hope this work will be helpful in improving mutual understanding and in strengthening further cooperation worldwide.

I have enjoyed preparing 'China's Sports Medicine' and deeply appreciate the colleagues who, through their knowledge and wisdom, have guided me. May this book fulfill its purpose.

Qu Mianyu, MD

Qu Mianyu, Yu Changlong (eds): China's Sports Medicine.
Medicine Sport Sci. Basel, Karger, 1988, vol 28, pp 1–6

Sports Medicine in China

Qu Mianyu

Institute of Sports Medicine, Beijing Medical University, Beijing, China

Therapeutic exercise as an important component of sports medicine is not something recent in China, it may be traced back as far as 2000 years ago. Examples include 'Daoyin' and 'Anqiao' (a kind of massage using both the hands and the feet) which were recorded in the famous old Chinese traditional medical book *Huan Di Nai Jing* produced in the Warring States Period (475–221 BC).

Daoyin, also called 'Xing Qi', is an exercise combining breathing exercises with movements made to imitate animals. Daoyin means keeping the vital energy going in harmony and making the body lithe. The stone inscribed 'On Xinqi' of the Warring States Period showed that methods of keeping and moving the vital energy were already known at that time. Monographs on Daoyin first appeared during the Western Han Dynasty (206–24 BC). A print on silk 'Daoyin Movement' unearthed in 1979 from the No. 3 Western Han Tomb in Changsha, Hunan province, is the earliest one discovered so far and the most complete picture of ancient gymnastics. The picture depicts, in color, 44 persons of different sex and age performing Daoyin exercises (fig. 1, 2). Doctor Hua Tuo (220–280 AD) of the period of the Three Kingdoms adapted some 40 Daoyin routines into five groups copied from the movements of the tiger, deer, bear, ape and bird, the so-called 'Wu Quin Xi' (5 animals exercise). During the Song Dynasty Daoyin was developed to 'Ban Duan Jin' which is still in vogue today (fig. 3). 'Yi Jin Jing' which came into being in the Ming (1368–1644 AD) and Qing (1644–1911 AD) dynasties combined breathing exercises and massage.

Daoyin is effective in prolonging one's life. The famous doctor San Simiao of the Tang Dynasty performed Daoyin exercises three times a day and died at the age of 110. Daoyin, therefore, was called in ancient times a 'longevity exercise'.

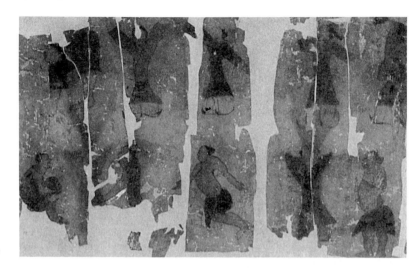

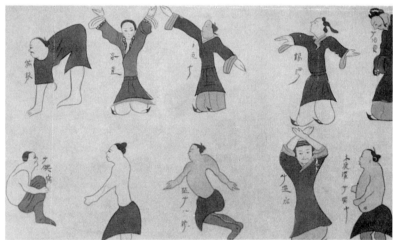

Fig. 1. 'Daoyin', painting on silk, unearthed from Western Han Dynasty (206 BD–24 AD) tombs at Mawangdui, Changsha, Hunan Province.

Fig. 2. The restored silk painting of 'Daoyin'.

In view of that mentioned above, it is easy to understand why some medical books of the western countries have called China the motherland of therapeutic exercise.

But as a comprehensive scientific subject and modern science, the age of sports medicine in China is still young, only about 30 years old.

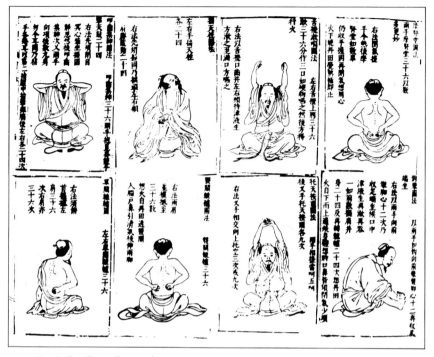

Fig. 3. Ban Dang Jin exercise.

China's sports have undergone several thousand years of development. But they had not been regarded as an undertaking of the state until 1949, when the new China was founded. Following the principles submitted by our government of popularizing sports among the people, enhancing their physique, and improving the sports skills of the country as a whole, a nationwide network for physical culture and sports as well as sports medicine and sciences has been set up and expenditure for these fields has been included in the state budget.

In 1958, the first orientation workshop of medical control of sport and therapeutic exercise was held in Beijing Medical College, directed by a professor from the USSR. In the meantime, similar workshops of sports physiology, anatomy and biochemistry have taken place at the Beijing Academy of Physical Culture and Sports. Also, the teaching of sports sciences has been built up throughout the country in medical and physical educational schools.

In 1958, the first research institute 'State Research Institute of Sports Science of Beijing' was established. It has divisions of sports medicine, medical control in sports, biochemistry, biomechanics, physiology and research laboratories for different sports events.

Just 1 year later, an independent research union of sports medicine named 'Beijing Research Institute of Sports Medicine' was set up in Beijing Medical College. Four research departments were developed: sports traumatology, sports nutrition and biochemistry, medical supervision, and rehabilitation.

Since then great achievement has been made in sports medicine in our country. Research institutes of sports science have been set up in 18 of 29 provinces, although serious disturbances have occurred during the 10-year period of internal derangement in our country.

It is only since The Third Plenary Session of the Eleventh Central Committee of the Chinese Communist Party, like other enterprises, under the guidance of restructuring and implementation of the opening-door policy to the outside world that sports medicine has taken a sound path and entered a new era. It has developed very quickly since then.

In 1978, the Chinese Association of Sports Medicine (CASM) was established, and accepted as a full national association member 2 years later (1980) by the FIMS (International Federation of Sports Medicine).

In 1980, CASM was fully established as one division of the Chinese Society of Sports Science, set up in 1980.

In 1983, the *Chinese Journal of Sports Medicine* was published. It is an important matter not only because of its influence in our country but also worldwide. About 34 countries have had an exchange programme with us, so it has also contributed worldwide in raising the academic standard of sports medicine.

Sports medicine in China now consists of several divisions: sports traumatology, medical supervision of sports, sports nutrition, sports rehabilitation, physiology, anatomy, biochemistry, and biomechanics concerning sports injury.

In regard to research work special attention has been attached to the following topics: (1) Determination of the physical ability for helping the coaches or the sport participants to make a sound exercise program by various functional evaluations. (2) Prevention and treatment of sports injuries and sports diseases. (3) Rehabilitation of sportsmen who are sick or injured. (4) Elimination of general fatigue by the proper use of nutrients, physical therapy, massage and Chinese traditional medicinal herbs. (5) Selection of athletes by comprehensive physical examination, bone age assessment, and determination of muscule fiber type and genetic factors. (6) Doping examination.

The research work must be connected closely to training work, and approaching the goal of *Health for All* has been emphasized by the government. There is a state research planning program submitted by the expert advisory commission led by the State Commission of Sports and Physical Culture. The state level research projects are mainly financed from the state budget. Research institutions may also have their own research subjects. In this case they must get support from the Ministry of Public Health and Ministry of Education or from various fundings in China or abroad.

At present, an overall research network has been established. This comprises research institutes of sports sciences (state level 1 and province level 18, under the direction of the Commission of Sports and Physical Culture), research institutes or labs of sports medicine in the medical schools, research union of sports science of the military, and departments of sports medicine, physiology, anatomy, biochemistry and biomechanics in the school of sports and physical culture. The research army has expanded a great deal in the recent 10 years, which is not only including the staff of researchers but also the rank of postgraduates. However, we still have problems of shortage of manpower, qualified researchers and modern equipment.

From 1953 to 1986 about 6000 articles were published. After the Third Plenary Session of the 11th Chinese Central Commission of the Chinese Communist Party, an estimated 800 papers concerning experimental or clinical studies were issued each year. The quality of the papers has also been raised a lot. Examples included research work on cartilage and tendon insertion injuries, chronic epihyseal injury, stress and fatigue fracture of the tibia and vertebral lamina, muscular strain and late soreness, treatment of exercise disease or elevating the physical ability of the athletes by using Chinese medicinal herbs, comprehensive functional evaluation particularly by the determination of lactic acid, special diet and drink for gymnastics and weight lifters, theoretical basis of 'Qi Gong' and gymnastic 'Tai ji', as well as Chinese massage for the treatment of chronic diseases and injuries and their usage in training, and prolonging life expectancy.

Since the establishment of CASM, all China scientific symposiums, meetings or conferences have been held on average twice a year; 1800 papers have been presented or published in poster form. Among them more than 50 were presented at international conferences or published in journals or books.

In 1985 'The Beijing International Conference of Sports Medicine' was held in Beijing. It may be an important historical matter in the development of sports medicine in China as well as the world.

Personally, as the vice president of the FIMS and the chairman of CASM, I sincerely hope the publication of *Sports Medicine in China*, will strengthen mutual understanding with other countries and develop further cooperation in raising the academic standard of sports medicine.

Qu Mianyu, MD, Institute of Sports Medicine, Beijing Medical University, Beijing (China)

Qu Mianyu, Yu Changlong (eds): China's Sports Medicine.
Medicine Sport Sci. Basel, Karger, 1988, vol 28, pp 7–18

Clinical and Pathological Studies on Enthesiopathy of Athletes

Qu Mianyu, Yu Changlong

Institute of Sports Medicine, Beijing Medical University, Beijing, China

Enthesiopathy, a degenerative lesion in tendon or ligament insertions caused by chronic strain, is one of the most common injuries in sports [1]. Examples include jumpers' knee, rotator cuff injuries [2], tennis elbow, painful syndrome of the hamstring tendon insertion on the ischium, and apophysitis. Although this kind of lesion is not severe, it is a 'technopathy' associated with a high incidence and difficulty in treatment, so for many years it has been an important topic in the field of sports medicine. This paper includes the normal structure of tendon or ligament insertion, pathology, pathogenesis, prevention and treatment of enthesiopathy, as investigated in our institute.

Normal Structure and Anatomical Classification of Tendon or Ligament Insertion [10]

Much of the literature published has been concerning the structure of the tendon insertion [Kollocker, 1852; Dolgo Saburoff, 1929; LaCava, 1952; Zwei Zuli, 1963]. Generally, it consists of five different structures: wavy fibers, fibrocartilage zone, tide line, calcified cartilage and bone. However, the function and the importance of subordinate structures have rarely been mentioned.

According to our experimental studies (in 2 groups of rabbits, the infrapatellar and Achilles tendon insertions were investigated individually) and clinical investigations of peritendinitis of the patellar and Achilles tendon, we found that although the main structures of tendon or ligament insertion are basically identical, the subordinate structures including the bursa, fat pad

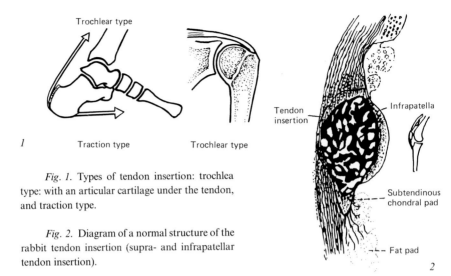

Fig. 1. Types of tendon insertion: trochlea type: with an articular cartilage under the tendon, and traction type.

Fig. 2. Diagram of a normal structure of the rabbit tendon insertion (supra- and infrapatellar tendon insertion).

and subtendinous chondral pad, are different based on their biological demands.

For example, the subtendinous chondral pad is found only in the patellar tendon insertion area, and various pathological changes could be found in the pad in peritendinitis of the patellar tendon. However, in the insertion of Achilles tendon, a layer of cartilage on the calcaneal tubercle just like the joint surface located opposite the tendon, functioning as a trochlea exists in place of the chondral pad. In this cartilage layer pathological changes in the enthesiopathy of Achilles tendon insertion could also be found. After a thorough study and comparison with the subordinate structures of tendon or ligament insertion in other parts of the body in humans and animals, a new concept for typing tendon or ligament insertions is submitted in this paper. Based on the variety of the subordinate structures, 3 types could be divided als follows:

(1) Trochlear type (e.g. rotator cuff, insertion of Achilles tendon): Characterized by a layer of cartilage located opposite to the tendon, functioning as a trochlea to increase the action force and decrease local friction between the tendon and bone (fig. 1).

(2) Bending traction type (e.g. Patellar tendon insertion): A special subtendon chondral pad under the attachment of the patellar tendon connected to the tip of the patella. Its special function is to decrease the traction force and prevent sharp angulation of the main structure of the insertion.

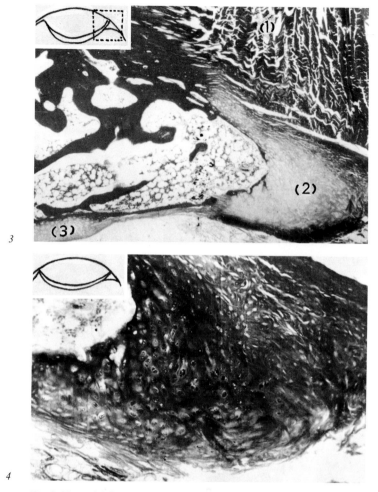

Fig. 3. Normal infrapatellar tendon insertion in rabbit. 1 = Tendon insertion (main); 2 = subtendon chondral pad; 3 = articular cartilage of the patella. Mallory stain, × 40.
Fig. 4. Subtendon chondral pad: rich glycogen granules in chondrocytes. PAS. × 100.

Schneider [6] and Becker [5] have pointed out that fiberocartilage in the main structure of insertion can prevent sharp angulation. But they did not mention the function of the special pad. Our contribution is to find out the special pad and its function, and define the bending-traction type of the insertion (fig. 2–5).

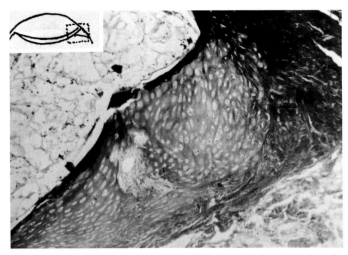

Fig. 5. Hydrocortisone injection group. Killed 12 weeks after 8 injections. Proliferation of connective tissue in the subtendon chondral pad. HE. × 100.

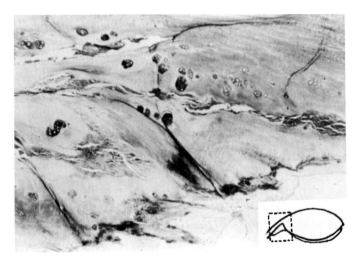

Fig. 6. Female, aged 63. Fibrocartilage zone: hyaline degeneration and chondrocyte island. Subtendon chondral pad: hyalinized and degenerated. PAS. × 160.

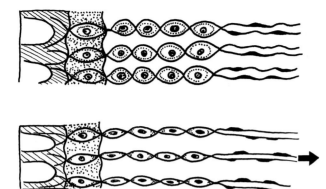

Fig. 7. Buffer function of different zones of the main tendon insertion during traction.

(3) Traction type (e.g. the insertion of plantaris aponeurosis in calcaneal bone): It mainly serves as a buffer to traction force. This type of insertion does not contain subordinate structures like cartilage surface or chondral pad beneath the tendon insertion except for the bursa (fig. 6).

Function of Tendon or Ligament Insertion

The main function of tendon or ligament insertion is to transmit a pulling force produced by the muscle to the working organ 'bone'. According to William's formula, traction force acting on the patellar tendon insertion is about 2–5 times body weight during the movement of the knee. As a buffer, the insertion makes the pulling force reduce gradually upon every unit area and avoids 'sudden action'. In general, this function is completed by the following factors:

(1) Wavy collagen and elastic fibers straighten during traction (fig. 7).

(2) Lacunae buffer: The lacunae of chondrocytes in the fibrocartilage zone change from round to spindle in shape during traction, it offers some extent of buffer (fig. 7).

(3) The matrix of fibrocartilage zone contains a considerable amount of glucosaminoglycan (GAG) which makes this zone work as a piece of rubber, changing its shape during bending and traction. We called it 'deformation buffer'. Some authors indicated that the calcified cartilage zone has a similiar function.

(4) Because the collagen fibers are embedded obliquely in bone, the area gets bigger along the direction from the tendon to the bone: the inser-

tion is just like a tree root, it reduces the pulling force acting upon every unit area.

(5) To reduce the bending stress by the subtendinous chondral pad.

(6) To reduce the stress by the cartilage surface under the rotator cuff or Achilles tendon by changing its thickness while the tendon is pulled and pressed on the cartilage surface (fig. 1, 8).

In view of that mentioned above, it is clear that for stress buffer, either the main or subordinate structure is the critical point and why both structures are easily injured.

Tendon insertion also has a function of increasing action force provided by the subtendinous chondral pad (patellar tendon) and trochlea (Achilles tendon or rotator cuff insertion), they make the levator arm increase.

Clinical Pathology and Aging Influence

Taking the peritendinitis of patellar tendon (painful apex type) as an example [4], 17 operated cases were studied clinically and pathologically. The findings are as follows:

(1) Tendon and peritendineum: The damaged area of tendon and peritendineum showed as being yellowish in color. Wavy arrangement of tendon fibers disappeared in mild cases. In severe cases, hyaline or fibrous degeneration usually existed. Fat tissue invasion, round cells infiltration and calcification was detectable in longitudinal section of the tendon. The peritendineum which contained more or less engorged, proliferated and sclerotic blood vessels became congested, edematous and firmly adherent to the tendon.

(2) Bone tissue: Fibrosis in the marrow cavity without osteoblastic proliferation. Marrow cavities opened somewhere toward the fibrocartilage zone of insertion.

(3) Fibrocartilage zone: Capillaries invaded into this area. In some cases, chondrocyte clumps just like hyaline cartilage cells were found in this area.

(4) Calcified cartilage became irregular in thickness. 'Microscopic avulsion fracture' was found in 1 case.

Aging Influence on the Patellar Tendon Insertion Area [13]

Fourteen specimens were collected at autopsy. Their age ranged from 1 to over 50. Among them, 1 day to 15, 4 cases; 16–49, 5 cases and over 50, 5 cases. After a thorough histological study on the patellar tendon insertion

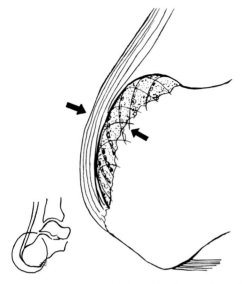

Fig. 8. Buffer function of the subtendon cartilage of Achilles tendon insertion. Trochlear type.

area of the different ages specimens, we found out that both the main and subordinate structures developed gradually and completely after birth in order to adapt to the physiological demand as buffer. This study also indicated that after 40, most cases revealed a definite degenerative change in tendon insertion as well as the subtendon chondral pad just like a typical enthesiopathy. Therefore, making a clinical diagnosis in the aging patient, if symptoms and signs existed, aging enthesiopathy should be considered instead of traumatic enthesiopathy.

Pathogenesis of Enthesiopathy

A series of experimental and clinical studies have been carried out for this purpose in our institute. They were: (1) An experimental study of enthesiopathy of rabbits' Achilles tendon [12]: 33 adult rabbits were used and divided into 3 groups:

(a) Control group: 5 rabbits were included. Specimens of Achilles tendon insertion region were studied histologically and histochemically. Among them 2 had angiography with Chinese ink through the abdominal aorta to study the local blood supply.

(b) Simple binding group (second control group): 28 rabbits were used. The position of binding was about 2 cm above the left ankle. Binding lasted 1.5 h daily for 2 or 4 weeks. Then the specimens were prepared for gross examination, X-ray, histological and histochemical examination (stained by HE, PAS, Mallory and Toluidine blue).

(c) Pulling and binding group: The remaining right legs of 28 rabbits were included. The leg was fixed on a table with a bandage, then flexed and extended passively by a specially designed motor traction unit, by which the insertion of the Achilles tendon sustained traction stress abruptly, repeatedly and rhythmically. Seventy-two times per minute, 1.5 h and totally 6,480 times of passive traction daily. As the second control group, 2 subgroups, 2 and 4 weeks, were set up. In each subgroup, rabbits were sacrificed in 3 different intervals, immediately after traction and 4 or 8 weeks rest after traction. Angiography was carried out in 16 of 28 rabbits with the same method as above. The specimens were treated in the same manner as in (a) and (b).

The results showed that either simple partial obstruction of venous return or passive traction force applied on Achilles tendon insertion could cause typical pathological changes of enthesiopathy. However, the changes caused by partial obstruction of venous return were more slight than by passive traction.

Having checked up the damages in the subordinate structure, it was so impressive that the damage was more severe than in the main structure, and its severity was closely related to the duration of traction. These pathological changes were: ectopic ossification in the fat pad, bursitis and hypertrophic change of the periosteum on the superior part of the calcaneal tubercle just near the margin of the subtendinous cartilage surface.

Therefore, we considered that a circulatory disturbance caused either by overloading or other factors as well as strain injury could be the etiological factor of enthesiopathy. We also suspected that the changes in subordinate structure might cause more severe symptoms than those in the main structure. When you examine a patient, do not forget to check the subordinate structure.

(2) We produced the animal model of epiphysitis on traction epiphysis (calcaneum) so-called 'apophysitis' on 64 young rabbits using the same method as above in order to investigate the pathogenesis and pathology [9].

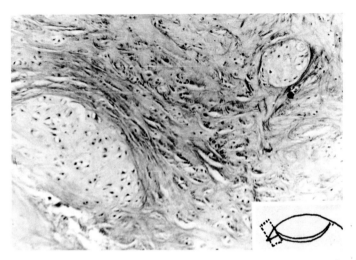

Fig. 9. Chondrofication (island formation) in the fibrocartilagenous zone of tendon insertion. HE. × 100.

Besides the changes on the epiphysis itself, we also found definite changes on the Achilles tendon insertion, both the main and subordinate structures. These changes proved that the enthesiopathy of Achilles tendon insertion also existed. So, in apophysitis, the pathological changes of enthesiopathy should be one part of the most important changes and should not be neglected.

On X-ray film of Osgood-Schlatter's disease, some authors thought the bone shadow in the patellar tendon is 'avulsion fracture'. We do not agree with this, it could be an ossification of the condral island after degeneration of the tendon (fig. 9).

(3) A group of rabbits was used to study the healing process of the articular surface after total excision of the patellar joint surface. It showed that during incomplete remodeling of the articular surface by new growing granulation tissue, osteoarthritis took place, accompanied by typical changes of enthesiopathy in the insertion of the extensor mechanism around the margin of the patella and formation of ossification or osteopathy in the capsule [8]. This indicated that after the normal relation between joint surfaces is destroyed, there might be some traumatic factors acting upon the insertion area and causing enthesiopathy.

Clinically, in the treatment of chondromalacia of the patella by patellectomy, we also noted that enthesiopathic changes in the insertion of the extensor mechanism existed. Its severity was closely related to the damage of the articular surface.

The reason for chondrofication or ossification in the tendon is still not clear. It has been proved in our work that chondrocytes in vitro, after 4–5 passages, would change the biological property from chondrocyte to fibrocyte. This phenomenon is 'dedifferentiation'. We also proved that from the bottom of a fresh articular defect the growing new granulation tissue could form a new fibrous articular cartilagenous surface gradually. This mechanism is 'metaplasia', induced by mechanical sliding irritation on the articular surface. Is there any relation between dedifferentiation and metaplasia? Under which kind of condition, the chondrocyte changes into a fibrocyte and vice versa remains unclear, further basic research is undoubtedly needed [11].

Treatment and Prevention

In this paper, we emphasized that for treatment and prevention of enthesiopathy in athletes, the anatomical characteristics of different types of insertion including main and subordinate structures should always be paid attention to, especially the subordinate structure. In conservative treatment, the most common methods are massage, physical therapy and local infiltration with various kinds of cortical steroid or nonsteroid drugs. However, abuse of drug infiltration should be avoided. In general, no more than 3 times injection is suitable, otherwise the drug will also cause degeneration or necrosis in the insertion area. This has been proved in another experiment by local injection of hydrocortisone, hyaluronidase, and Dan san solution (a kind of Chinese herb). So, some medication could be one of the etiological factors of enthesiopathy [7, 10].

The principles for surgical treatment are: (1) release tension in damaged insertion; (2) excision of inflamed bursa, severe degenerative tendon, etc.; (3) excision of adherent peritendineum and other adherent surrounding tissue.

Setting up a proper rehabilitation program for the operated or injured patient is of great importance. How to avoid the insertion sustaining the highest load after surgery is the key to the success of treatment. In a sense, it is also the key point for the prevention of enthesiopathy. For example, the Achilles tendon usually sustains much stress when the ankle is situated in a sharp angle, especially less than 70 of dorsal flexion, so this ankle position should be avoided when the patient jumps during the rehabilitation period.

Conclusions

(1) A new anatomical classification of tendon or ligament insertion is submitted in this paper according to anatomy and function of its main and subordinate structures. These are trachlea, traction and binding traction types.

(2) After 40 years of age, there are always some degenerative changes in the insertion area. Therefore, making the diagnosis of traumatic enthesiopathy should be done very carefully.

(3) Local circulatory disturbance, microtrauma and other acute or chronic traumatic factors could all be the etiological factors in enthesiopathy.

(4) In the treatment and prevention of enthesiopathy, the anatomical and biological characteristics of both the main and subordinate structures should always be noticed.

References

1   Qu Mianyu: Investigation about the treatment and prevention of sports injuries (an analysis of 2725 cases). J Beijing Med. Coll. 1965; 2:106.
2   Li Meijun, Qu Mianyu: Injury of rotator cuff in athletes. Symposium of National Congress of Sports Science. China Sports Editorial Board, 1964.
3   Qu Mianyu: An experiment pathological study of total excision of articular surface of the patella in rabbits. J Beijing Med. Coll. 1963; 4:275.
4   Qu Mianyu: Peritendinitis of the patellar tendon (patellar apex type). A collection of sports medicine; thesis Institute of Sports Medicine, Beijing Medical College, 1973, p 59.
5   Becker W, et al: Die Tendopathien. Stuttgart, Thieme, 1978.
6   Schneider H: Die Abnutzungserkrankungen der Sehnen und ihre Therapie. Stuttgart, Thieme, 1959.
7   Balasubramanian P, et al: The effect of injection of hydrocortisone into rabbit calcaneal tendon. J Bone Joint Surg 1982; 54B:729.
8   Qu Mianyu: Healing and regeneration of articular cartilage. An experimental and pathological study. Tainjin Orth 1964; 8 (suppl 1):5.
9   Wu Linsong, Qu Mianyu: Experimental study of chronic epiphyseal injury. Chinese J Sports Med. 1983; 2:13.

10 Qu Mianyu: Anatomical structure of patellar tendon insertion and local effect of drug injection. Biomechanics, Kinathropometry and Sports Medicine, Exercise Science (scientific program abstract). Eugene, 1984.

11 Yu Changlong, Qu Mianyu: Changes in biological properties of rabbits articular cartilage cells in vitro. Beijing Int. Conf. on Sports Medicine (abstract of paper). Beijing, 1985.

12 Yu Changlong, Qu Mianyu, et al: An experimental and pathological study on enthesiopathy of Achilles tendon insertion in rabbits. Symp of National Congr of Sports Science. China Sports Editorial Board, 1981.

13 Yu Changlong, Qu Mianyu: Anatomical structure of human patellar tendon insertion and its biological significance. J Beijing Med Coll 1983; 15:267.

Qu Mianyu, MD, Institute of Sports Medicine, Beijing Medical University, Beijing (China)

Qu Mianyu, Yu Changlong (eds): China's Sports Medicine.
Medicine Sport Sci. Basel, Karger, 1988, vol 28, pp 19–33

The Pathophysiology and Principles of Rehabilitation after Cartilage Injury

Qu Mianyu

Institute of Sports Medicine, Beijing Medical University, Beijing, China

Joint cartilage injuries, both acute and chronic, are extremely common occurrences in sports injuries. Some of them exist independently, such as chondromalacia of the patella or femoral trochlea but in the majority of cases they are accompanied by other injuries (such as rupture of knee ligaments or meniscus). The course of recovery is closely related to rehabilitative protocols which are based on the knowledge of the pathophysiology of cartilage injury.

For many years cartilage injury has been studied extensively in our institute, the pathogenesis, pathology of the repairing process and regeneration are the 3 areas in which we have concentrated our efforts. The experience we have gained shows great promise in treating cartilage injury cases. This paper is a summary of our experiences in this field and includes a brief review of the literature, which will establish a theoretical basis in planning a proper rehabilitative protocol.

The Normal Structure of Articular Cartilage

The normal joint surface has an amorphous superficial coating formed by mucous and fibrous layers. It has a wavelike appearance in rabbits when viewed under the scanning electron microscope. Beneath this layer, the real cartilage structure including chondrocytes, collagen and matrix is found (fig. 1).

According to Bennighoff [1925], the superficial collagen fibers arrange themselves tangentially, descending obliquely, and finally reaching a calcified cartilage layer and penetrating perpendicularly into the subcondral bone.

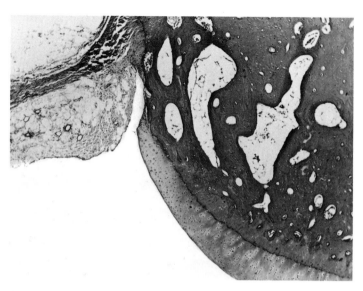

Fig. 1. Normal articular cartilage of patella in rabbit. HE. × 35.

Scattered chondrocytes arrange themselves along the fibers correspondingly. Based on the alignment of chondrocytes, cartilage could be divided into superficial, transitional, columnar, tide line and calcified layers.

Chondrocytes synthesize both the matrix and collagen. The matrix has a composition which is capable of binding water and it guarantees the mechanical properties of cartilage. It contains negatively charged polysaccharide molecules known as glucosaminoglycans (mucopolysaccharides, GAG), such as chondroitin 4 or 6 sulfate and keratin sulfate. When they attach to a protein core, the whole structure is called 'proteoglycan'. Normally, the degradation of GAG is balanced by the speed of synthesis. The half-life of GAG is from several days to a few months.

Chondrocytes contain lysosomes which can be broken down during cartilage injury and hemoarthrosis. Cathepsin D is then released which breaks down the proteoglycan. Proteoglycan can also be broken down by leukocyte enzymes at neutral pH.

Chondrocytes also synthesize collagen which is made up of 3 polypeptide chains in parallel spirals. The half-life of collagen is several months. Collagen fibers play an important role in maintaining the tensile strength of the articular cartilage. According to Curtis and Klin [1965], proteolytic enzyme cannot break down collagen in articular cartilage when the pH is around 7. During wound healing, a special enzymatic system denatures collagen and then normal collagen is vulnerable to attack.

Nutrition of Articular Cartilage

In order to maintain the normal structure of cartilage and its biochemical and mechanical functions, chondrocytes must maintain their metabolic function at a high level, thus sufficient nutrients are undoubtedly essential. These nutrients can be obtained in 2 ways:

(1) From the blood vessels of subchondral bone. This is only possible in growing individuals with open epiphyseal plates.

(2) From the blood vessels of the joint capsule. In adults, this is the only way to get nutrients from the body.

The synovial layer of the joint capsule has active function of secretion and absorption. Capillary loops exist in the synovial villi. Any change there could affect normal transportation in the capillaries. Synovial fluid contains glucose, electrolytes and low molecular weight protein which are transported into the joint cavity mainly by diffusion. In addition, there is hyaluronic acid which is made by the synovial cells.

Joint movement is the key to diffusion of nutrients from synovial fluid to cartilage and metabolites from cartilage to synovial fluid. Variations of pressure on the cartilage surface during joint movement works as a pump to help diffusion. Thus, normal blood supply, function of capillaries and joint movement are critical factors for the diffusion of substances between blood vessels and cartilage.

Changes in Articular Cartilage during Joint Movement

Morphology of Articular Cartilage Changes as Different Mechanical Stress Forces Act on the Joint Surfaces

Cotta and Pahl [9] showed that there are no collagen fibers to be seen histologically near the articular cartilage surfaces in the femoral condyle in rabbit embryo. On the other hand, many more cells, although not clearly classified into 4 zones, exist in the young embryo's cartilage. Postnatally, as mechanical stress forces on the joint surface increase, the cartilage surface gets much smoother and 4 zones can be distinguished clearly by morphology of chondrocytes histologically and histochemically. An extensive study on the human knee joint had similar findings. Morphological studies of articular cartilage also demonstrated that histological changes correspond with the changes of mechanical demands. The functions of chondrocytes including synthesis of collagen and matrix are no doubt changed as well. This fact reminds one that suddenly increased joint movement or mechanical stress (always happens in athletes owing to technical demand) could cause decomposition of cartilage and pathological change.

Immobilization of Joint (Including Compressive Fixation) Causes Degenerative Cartilage Changes

Bennighoff [1924], Freud [1937], Even [3], Salter and Field [4], and Trias [5] pointed out that when a joint is immobilized for an extended period, cartilage degeneration begins.

Lack of joint movement decreases the blood supply to the cartilage, fewer nutrients and oxygen move from capillary to cartilage by diffusion. Immobilization also causes connective tissue proliferation which blocks the path of diffusion. Long-term immobilization leads to imbalances in muscular tensile strength and then causes some joint regions to be continually compressed. These factors cause cartilage damage, possibly very serious damage.

In 1978, Refior[10] used a special device to fix rabbit knee and separate joint surfaces for the study of changes of cartilage after complete loss of joint movement and compression. After 4 months, pathological changes (very like osteoarthritis) had occurred in the joint cartilage.

Lack of Normal Physiological Irritation on the Articular Surface May Lead to Cartilage Damage

A group of rabbits were used for this purpose in our institute in 1966 [8]. Permanent dislocation of the patella was reproduced surgically on rabbits' knees. The results showed that a series of degenerative changes were present in the cartilage of the femoral condyle after a certain period following surgery. The cartilage got thinner, ossification began and blood vessel changes could be found. On the contrary, a new third femoral condyle developed, just opposite the dislocated patella, having a covering of a new and growing fibrocartilagenous articular surface. It is obvious that the new articular surface was due to the local mechanical irritation of the dislocated patella (fig. 2–4, 8–10).

These results indicated that normal irritation of cartilage provided by joint movement is necessary not only for the development of cartilage but

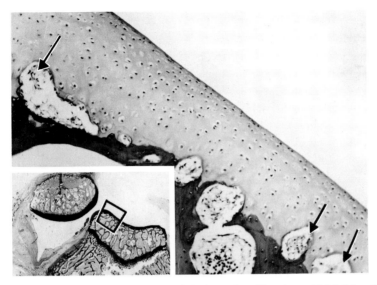

Fig. 2. Changes of articular cartilage of the femoral trochlea after artificial dislocation of the patella. Marrow cavity growing into the cartilage is shown. HE. × 100.

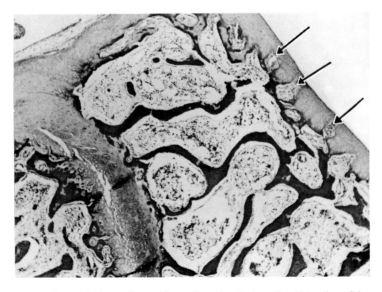

Fig. 3. Changes in the cartilage of femoral trochlea 15 days after dislocation of the patella. Thinning of the cartilage and marrow cavity growing in with fibrosis is revealed. HE. × 35.

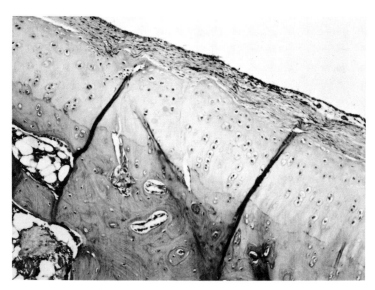

Fig. 4. 1.5 months after dislocation of the patella. Fibrous profliferation and fibrosis over the surface of the articular cartilage is seen. HE. × 100.

also for the maintenance of normal function of the joint articular cartilage surface. Lack of sufficient joint movement may cause degenerative changes in the cartilage. Therefore, a proper rehabilitative protocol is always needed after joint injury or disorders.

Rehabilitative Protocol Should Be Selected According to Pathology and Pathogenesis of Damaged Cartilage

Immobilization for a Long Period

Immobilization is harmful to muscles and cartilage. Although 'small splints' or specially designed metal braces have been used with good results in the treatment of a simple fracture of the limbs; however, in the treatment of complicated fractures, war injuries or ligament injuries as well as in ligament reconstruction, absolute immobilization of a joint is still necessary. So, which rehabilitative protocol is better to avoid the disadvantage caused by immobilization is worth finding out.

Böhler used to advocate a conservative method for treating acute knee ligament injuries. He said that even a long period of immobilization will not result in quartriceps atrophy when the patient can walk with a cast and perform isometric exercises. However, he did not mention if there was any cartilage injury in his patients. A number of arguments were raised after that. Our opinion is that Böhler's principle of rehabilitation should not be ignored completely. For those cases needing absolute immobilization, such as in transarticular fracture or ligament repair, his protocol could still be useful.

In 1976, Eriksson suggested the use of a special apparatus to partially immobilize the knee for 3 weeks after reconstruction of ACL. The knee still had movement (between 30 and 60). We were told that one half of the rehabilitation time could be saved by his method.

In 1978, Burri et al. [12] did three experiments in order to find a new rehabilitative protocol to be used after ligament reconstruction in the knee joints.

(1) Using knee joints from human amputation and cadaver, all ligaments were severed, then the ligaments were sutured with fine rubber threads to their original places. When any tension was placed on the ligament, the stretching of the rubber thread could reveal it clearly. The result revealed that no tension was placed on any of the four main ligaments when the knee was flexed from 20 to 60. However, any varus or valgus of the knee joint, rotation, or drawer test put great tension on them.

(2) In a second experiment, MCL, ACL of their knees were severed and sutured as above. Under controlled humidity conditions these knees were flexed 430000 times from 20 to 60, and no damage was found in the ligaments.

(3) The third experiment was done on animals. MCL of knees of ten rabbits were partially severed by one-third. After the operation, 5 rabbits' knees were allowed to move freely and the other 5 were immobilized in plaster casts for 3 weeks. Then the MCLs were examined and all were found to be fully healed. In the first 5 MCLs, fibroblasts and collagen were arranged in an orderly manner, but in the second group of 5, they lacked the normal layered arrangement.

These experiments revealed that active movement is feasible just after knee injury or surgery. However, according to our experiences this method is only theoretically feasible. If this method is used problems can occur. After a long immobilization, muscle atrophy causes the plaster cast to become loose thus losing effective immobilization. It is necessary to improve the techniques of immobilization.

In our institute, for cases needing long-term immobilization, we have used cotton splints underneath the plaster splints. This method has been used generally on more than 150 cases with ligament repair or reconstruction over 20 years. None had joint adhesions. The advantages of cotton splints are: (1) to stop bleeding by direct compression with cotton wadding which prevents articular cartilage damage from hemoarthrosis, and (2) in a thick cotton splint, the knee joint is still able to move through an angle of about 10; in addition, the extent of restraint could be controlled by the bandage (fig. 11).

If immobilization requests of the traction unit, such as in fractures of the tibial plateau or in complicated fracture of the elbow, arrangement must be made for some joint movement. This prevents joint adhesion. Also, joint movement could accellerate the change of granulation tissue on joint surface into cartilage.

Wear and Tear of Articular Cartilage [1]; its Influence on Sports Training and Related Rehabilitive Protocol

In the 1950s, a lot of young athletes in our country suffered knee and ankle pain, without any history of macrotrauma or positive X-ray change. Clinically, the physical examination and symptoms were very similar to chondromalacia or osteoarthritis due to age. The patients were unable to continue their training. Because of this, we began a clinical study and some other experiments in the early 1960s [6].

Firstly, an extensive medical survey was carried out in competitors in all sports. The results showed that the incidence of these chondromalacia- or osteoarthritis-like disorders was closely related to the techniques used in different sports such as 'footballer's ankle', one of the typical osteoarthrites of the ankle, which has a very high incidence in the football team.

Secondly, in order to study the pathogenesis of this kind of disorder and to prove that it is mainly due to overloading between articular surfaces, animal experiments were done using rabbits: (1) The rabbits' knees and ankles were moved against a 2 kg load passively by a specially designed motorized machine, working at 60 compressions per minute, 6 h per day and 6 days per week. (2) The rabbits' knees were extended by giving electric stimulations on the quardriceps in rhythm against resistance applied to foot, 60 stimulations per minute, 6 h per day, and 6 days per week.

Tissue specimens of knees and ankles were examined histologically and histochemically. Results showed that after 40 h of passive exercise of the joint, degenerative changes had started characterized by loss of chondroitin sulfate, local necrosis and presence of cell clusters in the cartilage.

This indicated that overuse of a joint by heavy striking or distortion between opposed articular cartilage can produce wear and tear of the articular cartilage. So, for a rehabilitative protocol in this kind of disorder, we have to: (1) give a suitable quantity and frequency of exercise as each case required; (2) do periodic movement first and then change to unperiodic movement when muscle strength recovers, and (3) never overwork or overmanipulate the joint to treat stiffness.

Hemoarthrosis and Joint Effusion

Intraarticular hemorrhage, either after trauma or associated with hemophilia, causes damage to the articular cartilage. This was proved in the animal by a few injections of their own blood [Dustmann, 1971].

Immobilization at the same time definitely increased the damage. It could be caused by either or both of the following;

(1) the changes of composition and density of synovial fluid may interfere with the normal diffusion between capsule and cartilage and (2) enzymes from the blood serum and blood leukocytes can cause enzymatic destruction of the superficial cartilage layer.

So, in these situations, before any rehabilitation can be begun, aspiration of the joint fluid or of blood should first be performed, then use of a heavy cotton splint with an elastic bandage to prevent a repeat of joint effusion. Finally, a selected rehabilitative protocol could be carried out.

In the case of septic arthritis, enzymes from bacteria and leukocytes cause severe and rapid destruction of the articular cartilage. We prefer to aspirate purulent fluid, then apply a skin traction to separate the cartilage surfaces and thus avoid compression on the joint surface caused by muscle spasm. Finally, the joint must be moved through its full range once a day for the prevention of joint adhesions.

Characteristics of the Repair Process after Cartilage Injury and Related Rehabilitative Protocol

In 1964, we performed experiments on rabbits dealing with the cartilage repairing process. Artificial damage including incision, superficial shaving and local cartilage defects with different depth were produced on the femoral

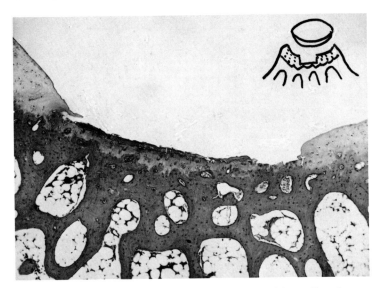

Fig. 5. Artificial cartilage defect reaching to the third layer of the cartilage shows no repair could be proven 5.5 months after surgery. HE. × 100.

condyle surfaces. Then, the tissue reactions were examined histologically and histochemically. The results showed that:

(1) After the superficial layer was excised, cartilage seemed to have the tendency to smooth the surface; however, the degenerative change existed permanently.

(2) Cartilage could not repair the damage going down into 2nd to 4th layers. However, cell proliferation was easily found around the damage (fig. 5).

(3) With cartilage damage going down into the subchondral bone, new growing granulation tissue could change metaplastically into hyaline-like cartilage. The defect could be repaired when mechanical stimulation was used (fig. 6, 7).

(4) When the cartilage defect extended down into the subchondral bone and there was no physiological mechanical stimulation, the new growing granulation tissue would not change to cartilage. This was proven by another of our experiments on rabbits. If the patellae were dislocated, the cartilage defect of femoral condyle would not be repaired metaplastically. This experiment also indicated that a local stimulation of the patella on the femoral

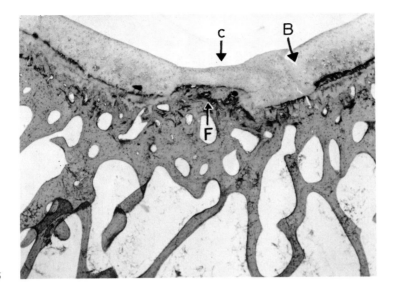

6

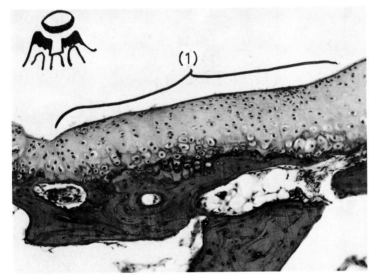

7

Fig. 6. Cartilage defect deep into the subchondral bone with the patella in the normal site, the new growing granulation changed metaplastically to fibrous cartilage 6 months after surgery. F = new growing subchondral bone; C = fibrous cartilage; B = margin of the artificial defect. HE. × 40.

Fig. 7. Newly growing hyaline-like cartilage repaired the defect at 6.5 months, when the patella is in the normal position and the defect is made deep into the subchondral bone. HE. × 100.

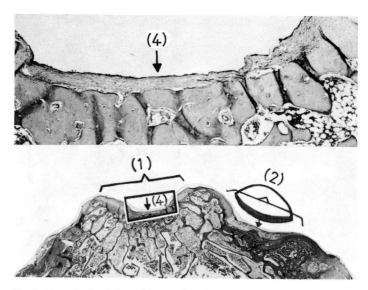

Fig. 8. Tissue in the defect of the cartilage is still fibrous in nature when the patella is dislocated for 1.5 months.

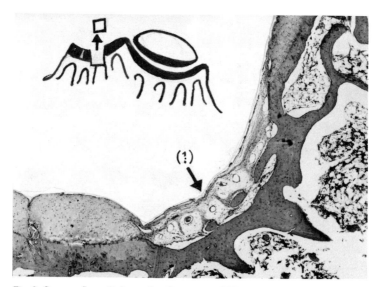

Fig. 9. Same as figure 8, 3 months after surgery. HE. × 35.

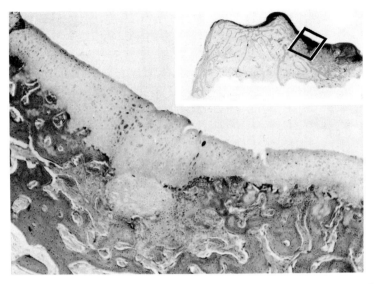

Fig. 10. Opposite to the dislocated patella a third condyle appeared with a new fibrous articular cartilage. HE. × 35.

condyle should start as early as possible and certainly never later than 2 weeks after the cartilage injury or operation (fig. 8, 9).

So, for successful rehabilitation, certain practices should be followed after cartilage injury.

(1) For wear and tear of cartilage, rehabilitation should avoid overwork or overload of the joint. Otherwise, new cartilage damage or chondral fracture will follow.

(2) For osteochondral fractures with hemoarthrosis, the blood in the joint cavity should be aspirated immediately and followed by compressive binding to prevent new bleeding. Movement of non-weight-bearing joints may start 10–14 days after the injury to enhance the metaplastic process. Approximately 6 months are needed to complete this repair process. This means that injured athletes can only be permitted to return to normal training 6 months after their injury.

(3) For joint chondropathy treated by surgical debridement, the principles of rehabilitation mentioned above should be followed, or the athlete will never be physically able to return to strenuous training.

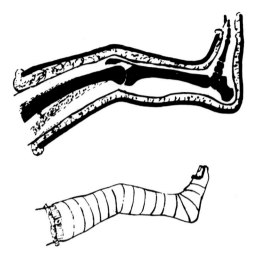

Fig. 11. A thick cotton splint with anterior and posterior plaster splints can provide 10°
movement (flexion and extension) during fixation.

Significance of Contact Area of Articular Surfaces for Rehabilitation

Let us take the knee joint as an example. During knee movement, the
patella moves along the femoral trochlea. So, at different knee angles, there
are different contact areas between the patella and the femoral trochlea. We
prefer to divide them into 30, 60, 90 and 120 areas. Clinically, symptoms and
signs existing at a certain angle always mean that the area is injured. We
could use this to plan our rehabilitative protocol. The patient information
would: (1) raise the straight leg against resistance; (2) do semisquatting static
exercise at a nonpainful angle (this method is routinely used in treatment of
patello-femoral joint chondropathy and in simple chondromalacia of the
patella): it is an isometric exercise; (3) do isokinetic or isotonic exercises
including concentric or eccentric exercise at a nonpainful angle to improve
muscle strength.

Another example is the joint contact surfaces between the femoral tibial
joint. The articular surface of the tibial plateau can be divided into 2 different
areas: the periphery, covered by a meniscus, and the center which is not
covered. It was reported that the structure of cartilage of these two parts is
different. After meniscectomy, we cannot start therapeutic exercise too
quickly, because it takes time for the structure on the peripheral area to
reform.

References

1 Barnett CH: Wear and tear in joint. J Bone Joint Surg 1956; 38B: 567.
2 Eichelberg L: Biochemical studies of articular cartilage, 111 values following immobilization of extremity. J Bone Joint Surg 1964; 41A: 1127.
3 Even EB: Experimental immobilization and remobilization of rat knee joint. J Bone Joint Surg 1960; 42A: 737.
4 Salter RB, Field P: Effect of continuous compression on living articular cartilage. J Bone Joint Surg 1960; 42A: 31.
5 Trias A: Effect of persistent pressure on articular cartilage. J Bone Joint Surg 1961; 43B: 376.
6 Qu Mianyu, et al: An experimental study of wear and tear of articular cartilage. Chinese Surg J 1963; 11: 339.
7 Qu Mianyu et al: Healing and regeneration of the articular cartilage. An experimental and pathological study. Tianjin Orth 1964; 8(suppl): 5.
8 Qu Mianyu, et al: An experimental study of the mechanical effects on the healing and regenerative process of injured articular cartilage. J Beijing Med College 1966; 2: 127.
9 Cotta H, Puhl W: The pathophysiology of damage to articular cartilage. Prog Orth Surg 1978; 3: 15.
10 Refior HJ, Hackenbroch MH. Jr: The reaction of articular cartilage to pressure, immobilization and distraction. Prog Orth Surg 1978; 3: 54.
11 Ruter A, Burri C: Retropatellar cartilage degeneration: diagnosis and outline of treatment. Prog Orth Surg 1978; 3: 143.
12 Burri C, Helbing, Spier W: The rehabilitation of knee ligament injuries. Prog Orth Surg 1978; 3: 54.

Qu Mianyu, MD, Institute of Sports Medicine, Beijing Medical University, Beijing (China)

Qu Mianyu, Yu Changlong (eds): China's Sports Medicine.
Medicine Sport Sci. Basel, Karger, 1988, vol 28, pp 34–42

Long-Term Follow-Up Study of Abnormal Electrocardiograms in Athletes

Gao Yunqiu, Pu Junzong, Zhang Baohui

Institute of Sports Medicine, Beijing Medical University, Beijing, China

It is now routine for the physician to include an electrocardiogram in the periodic health examination of asymptomatic people. It forms part of the regular health examinations of sports persons, particularly those engaged in endurance training. In athletes, the so-called 'abnormal' electrocardiogram is assessed as an isolated finding without the support of confirmatory evidence. Because the suspicion of heart disease may have a far-reaching effect upon the athletes, it is important to identify beyond any reasonable doubt the clinical significance of those variants that appear in the electrocardiograms of apparently healthy people.

In sports cardiology, certain physiopathological aspects, particularly electrocardiographic aspects, are still open to research [1]. This problem was brought clearly into focus in sports medicine when examples of atrioventricular heart block, right bundle branch block, variety of unusual T wave changes and some others were found in the routine electrocardiograms of some apparently healthy well-trained athletes [2]. Similar experiences were reported elsewhere [3]. More urgent matters required attention at that time but it was clear that a long-term follow-up study would be necessary to show the delayed effects of exercise on future cardiovascular events.

It is the purpose of this report to evaluate the abnormal electrocardiograms in athletes during their active training period and, after cessation of physical activities, present the results of medical examinations recorded between the years 1958 and 1972.

Material and Method

Subjects included 119 athletes, 94 male, 25 female, who have had certain electrocardiographic abnormalities. A follow-up study of 10–25 years was performed. At their last examination all the athletes had already ceased the strenuous training and their physical activity was lowered. The majority of the athletes had only one electrocardiographic abnormality and the others had more than one.

Medical examination included past history and present illness, physical examination, electrocardiogram at rest and chest X-ray. Laboratory test, echocardiogram, exercise stress test, Holter electrocardiogram, cardiac output, and stroke volume were performed when necessary.

Results and Discussion

The electrocardiographic changes during the follow-up period were as shown in table I.

II A-V Block

II A-V block is a very uncommon finding in normal people, but is significantly more frequent in young athletes and physically active middle-aged persons. After quite a long period of investigation by many authors, these blocks have been attributed to the absolute or relative increase of resting vagal tone following physical training and therefore these have been regarded as physiological phenomena. More than 80 athletes with II A-V block were observed and most of them were active, fit and had no complaints, only a few related to overstress, overfatigue or infectious diseases. It is believed that the majority of the II A-V blocks in athletes are functional blocks. This view has been questioned by Young et al. [4] who observed in 7 of 16 adolescents and adults a progressive worsening of A-V conduction up to fixed complete heart block, some of them even needed a pacemaker to live. The author also pointed out that neither a positive response to exercise and atropine nor the results of the electrophysiological investigation can be considered reliable prognostic indices. In 1980, Zeppilli et al. [5] revisited this old problem and reported 10 athletes, completed a noninvasive protocol study consisting of reflex autonomic tests, autonomic drug administration and physical exercise, 6 cases were followed up for 1.5–6 years, after cessation of training II A-V blocks vanished, no symptoms. The author believed that this event can still be considered a vagally-induced benign feature of athletes' heart. The clinical histories of these athletes and the observed complete disappearance of conduction disturbances after detraining strongly support

Table I. ECG changes during the follow-up period

Variant	Number	Unchanged	Diminished	Worsened	Disappeared
II A-V B	18	–	–	–	18
III A-V B	1	1	–	–	–
IRBBB	43	5	28	5	5
RBBB	9	9	–	–	–
T changes	27	4	14	6	3
PB	24	–	4	–	20
PT	4	–	–	–	4
WPW	5	4	–	–	1
LAH	3	3	–	–	–
RAR	3	1	–	–	2
LAR	1	–	–	–	1
JE	4	1	–	–	3
JR	4	–	–	–	4
VR	1	–	–	–	1

Abbr.: A-V B = Atrioventricular block; IRBBB = incomplete right bundle branch block; PB = premature beat; PT = paroxysmal tachycardia; WPW = Wolff-Parkinson-White; RAR = right atrial rhythm; JE = junctional escape; JR = junctional rhythm; VR = ventricular rhythm.

this opinion. Recently, 29 Japanese athletes were described, 15 cases were followed up for 2 weeks to 17 years, none developed III A-V block and the II A-V blocks were changeable. One athlete who was followed up for 17 years was an outstanding runner, after cessation of training II A-V block disappeared. Most of the II A-V blocks were caused by vagotonia, overfatigue in 2, overstress in 2, suspicious infectious disease in 1, and unknown in 2. The majority of the II A-V blocks are physiological changes and the prognosis is good [6].

In this study 18 elite athletes, 15 male, 3 female, have been followed up for more than 10 years, and 14 of the 18 for more than 20 years. At last examination II A-V blocks disappeared and electrocardiogram showed normal in 13, I A-V block in 3, RBBB in 1 and nonspecific T wave change in 1. The athletes have stopped training for many years, all are in good health and have no evidence of heart diseases.

III A-V Block

III A-V block is very rare in athletes. A female swimmer with a III A-V block followed up for 10 years who led a normal life and work including physical performance of many sports events has been presented in a previous paper. During follow-up her heart was slightly enlarged and she had a syncopal attack once with loss of consciousness for a few seconds. Though echocardiogram and exercise stress test were normal, cardiomyopathy could not be ruled out [7]. Hanne-Paparo et al. [8] reported a similar case, a soccer player with complete heart block who was asymptomatic and had never had complaints such as fatigue, dizziness or syncope. The author also reviewed the literature, and summarized that most patients with complete heart block without structural heart disease develop normally and have a normal physical capacity. If there are no Adams-Stokes attacks and high grades of ectopy at rest and at exercise, they can perform normal day-to-day tasks including strenuous work and sports.

IRBBB

Seventeen cases were followed up for more than 20 years. The majority of the IRBBB are changeable. Among the worsened 5 cases, 2 developed RBBB who had suspicious heart disease (CHD), 3 still showed an IRBBB pattern, 1 of the 3 had paroxysmal atrial fibrillation and 2 are healthy. Murayama et al. [9] found that IRBBB is reversible, and reported 88 cases of Japanese Olympic athletes who had IRBBB; 12 years later, 50% of the IRBBB disappeared after cessation of training, but it took longer to reduce than I and II A-V block. The animal experiment of Moore et al. [10] showed that IRBBB is related to right ventricular hypertrophy, there were no conduction system abnormalities in the right ventricle. So, IRBBB may be an electrocardiographic misnomer. From the genesis and development of IRBBBs, part of them may be related to physical training. Nowadays, many sports doctors believe that there is no restriction on joining physical training and competition. It should be taken into consideration that IRBBB developed into RBBB in a few cases.

RBBB

Massing et al. [11] reported 59 cases of acquired RBBB. When first diagnosed the cause of RBBB was unknown and the follow-up period was 4.5 years on average, the longest being 19 years. At the last examination only 1 person had CHD symptoms who had had hypertension on entry and others had good prognosis. Mathewson et al. [12] reported 30 cases from an apparently healthy population pertaining to 3,987 military and civilian pilots with a follow-up period of 10.6 years, all remained in apparent good health with 2 exceptions who died of noncardiac causes. Rotman et al. [13] reported

372 cases, the majority of whom had no symptoms at first examination, only 3% showed evidence of CHD, 2% had hypertension and after 10.8 years 14 died, 2 of myocardial infarction, 1 of cor pulmonale, and the others of noncardiac causes. The previous literature has shown that the prognosis of isloated RBBB without associated cardiovascular diseases is always good. In this study 6 of the 9 cases were followed up for more than 20 years. Three cases are believed to be of congenital origin, all are in good health and the RBBB pattern persisted. Six cases were acquired RBBB, 2 from IRBBB and 4 from normal electrocardiogram changed for RBBB, 3 are in good health and 3 had cardiac symptoms. Among the latter, 2 had clinically diagnosable CHD, 1 died suddenly at the age of 51, the other was suspected of having CHD.

T Wave Changes

The follow-up period exceeded 20 years in 10 athletes. Three cases showed giant T wave inversion. One had CHD whose T wave improved and 3 had suspicious CHD, T wave improved in 2 and worsened in 1.

There are different opinions about giant T wave inversion in the literature. Piovano et al. [14] considered 2 athletes with giant T wave inversion as having pathological left ventricular hypertrophy, as the electrocardiogram worsened after exercise and they joined some sports in which the cardiovascular system was less stressed. Nishimura et al. [15] published 6 cyclists with a follow-up period of 5 years, electrocardiogram worsened in 5 and persisted in 1. It was related to left ventricular hypertrophy, probably caused by prolonged strenuous training and seemed not to be caused by CHD. Kanoh et al. [16] found that giant T wave inversion among cyclists is related to apex cardiomyopathy, whether it was caused by an inner factor or by prolonged physical training could not yet be settled. Recently, hypertrophic cardiomyopathy associated with T wave change came into consideration, it is a cause of sudden death among young athletes [17].

On the other hand, Venerando et al. [18] reported giant T wave inversion in 15 well-trained athletes, followed up for 5–26 years, whose electrocardiogram showed 7 characteristics, no pathologic development, and no pathological significance. Rost et al. [19] are not aware of any case in the literature with ST-T change in which an invasive investigation including coronagraphy unveiled a cardiac disease, except for the case of Friok who found myocardial damage by echocardiography and myocardial scintigram. In this study 3 athletes with giant T wave inversion had normal echocardiogram and the inverted T improved after cessation of training. As the giant T wave inversion improved after cessation of training with normal echocardiogram and no signs of cardiac hypertrophy, exercise training might be one of the causative factors of its development. This problem needs further study. These modifications cannot generally be interpreted as pathologic or signs of overtraining. An invasive clinical investigation does not seem to be justified. Hypertrophic cardiomyopathy should be especially carefully excluded by echocardiogram. Under these preconditions a continuation of training can be permitted.

Premature Beat

Twenty-four athletes were surveyed. There was ventricular premature beat in 17, atrial in 6, junctional in 1, and frequent beats in 14, some forming bigeminy or trigeminy. At last examination the premature beats disappeared in 10 and were diminished in 4. There were 10 occasional premature beats, all of which disappeared. During follow-up, 3 cases had paroxymal atrial fibrillation, among them 2 had suspicious CHD and 1 is in good health. One who had occasional premature beat had clinically diagnosed CHD.

It is commonly known that premature beat belongs to unimportant changes. Mathewson et al. [12] stated that whether people with premature beat develop more serious arrhythmia or not has not yet been settled. In this study, most premature beats disappeared or diminished, the athletes' health conditions were good even with frequent premature beats forming bigeminy and trigeminy, only a few athletes had serious arrhythmia and CHD.

Paroxysmal Tachycardia

Ventricular tachycardia (1 case) and supraventricular tachycardia (3 cases) were provoked by overfatigue, after recovery from overfatigue there were no more paroxysms, all cases are healthy and there is no evidence of heart disease. In the previous literature many authors reported paroxysmal ventricular tachycardia that may occur in the absence of underlying organic heart diseases. It is, however, a relatively uncommon disorder [20].

Wolff-Parkinson-White Syndrome

Type A, 3 cases, 1 disappeared, 2 persisted and type James 2 persisted, all were healthy and no heart diseases were diagnosed. Attacks of paroxysmal tachycardia was provoked by intensive training in 2 athletes, during the attacks physical performance was negatively influenced and their life spans were reduced.

Left Anterior Hemiblock (LAH)

The electrocardiographic changes persisted and the athletes remained in good health. Wang et al. [21] reported 5 athletes with LAH, immediately after exercise LAH was unchanged, they pointed out that if LAH still persists with no signs of improvement, a pathological change could not be excluded. This remains to be verified.

Right Atrial Rhythm

The electrocardiographic signs disappeared in 2 and persisted in 1 case, in whom they vanished immediately after exercise and reappeared later. The athletes were healthy.

Left Atrial Rhythm

An elite male swimmer had left atrial rhythm when he was 19 years old which disappeared soon after, but 10 years after cessation of training, serious arrhythmia appeared including atrial premature beat, atrial fibrillation, atrial flutter, paroxysmal tachycardia, and enlarged heart with clinical symptoms. A diagnosis of cardiomyopathy was made.

Junctional Escape

The electrocardiographic features disappeared in 3 cases, persisted in 1, and the athletes are all healthy.

Junctional Rhythm

The abnormal rhythm existed temporarily. One of the athletes had hypertension.

Ventricular Rhythm

One athlete with temporary ventricular rhythm remained in good health.

Conclusions

II A-V block, IRBBB, paroxysmal tachycardia, premature beat, T wave change, junctional escape, junctional rhythm, ventricular rhythm and right atrial rhythm are related to physical training and tend to occur intermittently, while left anterior hemiblock, WPW syndrome, RBBB, III A-V block and left atrial rhythm usually remained constant once they appeared. The majority of the athletes were in good health and only a few showed evidence of cardiovascular disease. The prognosis of the athletes with abnormal electrocardiograms is determined by the presence or absence and degree of associated cardiovascular diseases, not the abnormal electrocardiograms themselves.

Summary

One hundred and nineteen athletes with abnormal ECGs were followed for over 10 years with an average of 17.5 ± 5.09 years, the longest for 25 years. II A-V B, IRBBB, paroxysmal tachycardia, premature beat, T wave change, junctional escape and rhythm, ventricular rhythm, and right atrial rhythm, in most athletes, was related to physical training and tended to occur intermittently, while left anterior hemiblock, WPW, RBBB, III A-V B and left atrial rhythm usually remained constant once they appeared. The majority of the athletes were in good health and only a few had evidence of cardiovascular disease. CHD (2.5%, 1 case died suddenly = 0.8%), suspicious CHD (5%), cardiomyopathy (1.7%), hypertention (0.8%), and paroxysmal atrial fibrillation (5%) were diagnosed. The prognosis of the athletes with abnormal ECGs is determined by the presence or absence and degree of associated cardiovascular diseases, not the electrocardiographic changes themselves.

References

1   Masini V: Concluding remarks; in Sports Cardiology, Bologna, Aulo Gaggi, 1980; pp 693–696.
2   Gao YQ, et al: Evaluation of athletes electrocardiogram. Sports Sci 1982; 1:51–57.
3   Venerando A: Electrocardiography in sports medicine. J Sports Med 1979; 19:107–128.
4   Young D, et al: Wenckebach atrioventricular block (Mobitz type I) in children and adolescents. Am J Cardiol 1977; 40:393–399.
5   Zeppilli P, et al: Wenckebach second-degree A-V block in top-ranking athletes: an old problem revisited. Am Heart J 1980; 100:281–294.
6   Gao YQ, et al: II A-V block in Japanese athletes. Chin J Sports Med 1985; 4:167–169.
7   Gao YQ, et al: Complete heart block and physical exercise. Chin J Sports Med 1987; 6:91–96.
8   Hanne-Paparo N, et al: Complete heart block and physical performance. Int J Sports Med 1983; 3:9–13.
9   Murayama M, et al: Cardiovascular future of athletes. J Phys Fitness Jpn 1980; 29:117–123.
10 Moore EN, et al: Incomplete right bundle-branch block. An electrocardiographic enigma and possible misnomer. Circulation 1971; 44:678–687.
11 Massing GK, et al: Clinical significance of acquired RBBB in 59 patients without overt cardiac disease. Aerospace Med 1967; 40:967–971.
12 Mathewson FAL, et al: Abnormal electrocardiograms in apparently healthy people. I. Long term follow-up study. Circulation 1960; 21:196–203.

13 Rotman M, et al: A clinical and follow-up study of right and left bundle branch block. Circulation 1975; 51:477–484.

14 Piovano G, et al: Frequency of ECG abnormalities in athletes. A study of 12,000 ECGs; in Sports Cardiology. Bologna, Aulo Gaggi, 1980, pp 625–630.

15 Nishimura T, et al: Noninvasive assessment of T-wave abnormalities on precordial electro-cardiograms in middle-aged professional bicyclists, J Electrocardiol. 1981; 14:357–364.

16 Kanoh T, et al: Myocardial hypertrophy associated with giant T wave inversion. J Clin Exp Med 1978; 105:623–636.

17 Maron BJ, et al: Sudden death in young athletes. Circulation 1980; 62:218–229.

18 Venerando A, et al: Anomalies of ventricular repolarization in athletes. A long term follow-up study. XXth Wld Congr Sports Medicine, Congr Proce, FIMS, Australia 1974, p 517.

19 Rost R, et al: Athletes' heart. A review of its historical assessment and new aspects. Int J Sports Med 1983; 4:147–165.

20 Gao YQ, et al: Paroxysmal ventricular tachycardia in athletes without organic heart dis-ease. Chin J Sports Med 1986; 5:88–92.

21 Wang GY, et al: A primary analysis on the electrocardiogram of left anterior hemiblock in athletes. Chin J Sports Med 1984; 3:193–195.

Gao Yunqiu, MD, Institute of Sports Medicine, Beijing Medical University,
Beijing 100083 (China)

Qu Mianyu, Yu Changlong (eds): China's Sports Medicine.
Medicine Sport Sci. Basel, Karger, 1988, vol 28, pp 43–51

Exercise-Induced Urinary Abnormalities in Athletes

Pu Junzong

Institute of Sports Medicine, Beijing Medical University, Beijing, China

There have been a number of reports dealing with urinary abnormalities after exercise [15], but these have usually been case reports [36]. On the basis of clinical observation and research work over several years, the exercise-induced urinary abnormalities in athletes were analyzed. The purpose of this study is to analyze the different types of urinary abnormalities after exercise and their associated clinical features, so as to provide a basis for diagnosis and management.

The training-related features which would influence the urinary abnormalities after exercise are as follows:

(1) Sport events. Many authors found that long-distance runners, soccer players, and basketball players have a much higher incidence of exercise-induced urinary abnormalities than gymnasts and weightlifters. Poortmans [27] has documented the same correlation, but the cause of the phenomenon was not defined.

(2) Intensity of training: In general, the incidence of urinary abnormalities after exercise is proportional to the severity of exercise [10]. When the subject is not yet adapted to the early phase of hard-training, urinary protein excretion after training appears in large amounts. With certain periods of persistent training, under the same workload, the protein excretion is significantly decreased.

(3) Environmental influence: Temperature and altitude have a significant influence on exercise-induced responses [34]. After swimming in very cold water the incidence and amount of excretion of urinary protein is much higher than after swimming at ordinary temperature. It has been documented that physical training at a high altitude had a higher incidence of proteinuria and hematuria than that at sea level.

(4) Constitutional factors: We have observed that urinary protein excretion and appearance of exercise hematuria have a great individual variation. One of the possible causes is related to the constitution of the subject. Liljefors [1969] had also noted that constitution played an important role in the exercise-related urinary abnormalities.

The types of the exercise-induced urinary abnormalities are varied, but mainly related to five types of urinary findings: exercise proteinuria, exercise hematuria, exertional hemoglobinuria, exercise cylindruria, and exertional myoglobinuria.

Table I. Incidence of proteinuria in different events of sport (compiled from Chinese reports) [32]

Sport event	Number of subjects	Sex	After race	After training	Year of report
Marathon	26	M	50–300 (76.9)		1985
Marathon	30	M	5–150 (97.0)		1975
Marathon	11	M	5–110 (64.0)		1973
Marathon	12	M	71.0 (100.0)		1964
Long-distance race	71	M	(80.4)		1964
Weight lifting		M	10–45		1962
Shooting	147		(43.0)		1962
Gymnastics	8		75 (89.0)	60 (66.0)	1961
Soccer		M	30 (90.0)	41 (43.0)	1963
Basketball			39.6 (88.4)	0–20 (15.0)	1963
Badminton	35		36.6 (68.4)	5.5 (21.2)	1964
Adolescent sprint	118			(74.8)	1963
Adolescent distance race	103			(63.0)	1963
100 m swim			31.8 (96.0)	31.0 (83.3)	1964
200 m swim			46.2 (100.0)		1964
Long-distance swim	19	F	41 (79.0)		1963
Speed skating	19	F	51.1 (100.0)		1964
Speed skating	18	M	35.1 (100.0)		1964
Long-distance skating	19	F	30.0 (89.5)		1964
Long-distance skating	16	M	25.9 (62.5)		1964
50 km bicycling	9		68.3 (88.9)		1965
100 km bicycling	12		25–100 (66.6)		1965

Excretion of urinary protein in mg%: incidence rate in parentheses.

Exercise Proteinuria

It has been known from the last century that urinary protein excretion increases after physical exercise. The German scientist von Leube [1877] found proteinuria after march and battalion training. After that, the terms such as 'physiological proteinuria', 'benign albuminuria' and 'exercise proteinuria' have been used widely. The incidence of proteinuria varied in different reports (table I).

In general, protein excretion reached the peak level in 20–30 min after exercise; albumin usually disappeared from the urine within 24 h sometimes 48 h. Urinary excretion in 72 subjects of different ages is shown in table II. In young distance runners the amount of protein excretion varied from 5 to 480 mg (average 123.5 ± 14.2 mg). In the young marathon runners protein excretion varied from 5 to 200 mg (average 48.5 ± 26.3 mg). In middle-aged subjects protein excretion varied from 5 to 160 mg (average 63.2 ± 16.3 mg). The results showed that appearance of proteinuria after exercise is closely related with exercise intensity. In the early stage of the study, exercise-induced proteinuria was found mainly in the form of albumin and has the same appearance as that from renal disease [27].

Examination of urinary protein by electrophoresis and immunological methods found that the major part of the content belongs components of plasma origin [McKay, 1962; Poortmans, 1962]. Recently, it was documented that the exercise proteinuria seems to be a mixed glomerulotubular type, the former being predominant [28]. The mechanism of exercise proteinuria is still unclear and there is no general agreement on the nature of the protein excretion. Because the urinary protein presented albumin, transferrin, IgG, haptoglobin type 2-1, increased glomerular permeability was suggested [26].

Table II. Urinary protein excretion in different age of athletes

Event of sport	Number of subjects	Age	Urinary protein excretion				
			below 10	11– 50	51– 100	101– 200	over 300
Long-distance race	18	20.2 ± 1.9	2	6	4	3	2
Marathon	20	22.2 ± 2.7	14	4		2	
Long-distance race	20	58.9 ± 9.0	8	5	5	2	
Marathon	14	62.3 ± 3.9	5	5	2	2	

Table III. The diagnosis in 112 cases of athlete's hematuria

Diagnosis	Male	Female	Total	%
Exercise hematuria	49	6	55	49.1
Glomerulonephritis	9	9	18	16.0
Urinary stones	13	3	16	14.3
Infection of urinary tract	2	11	13	11.7
Contusion of kidney	3	1	4	3.6
Exertional hemoglobinuria with hematuria	2	0	2	1.8
Congenital anomaly of kidney	1	0	1	.9
Idiopathic hematuria	1	0	1	.9
Hydronephrosis	1	0	1	.9

The mechanism of this increase may be explained by several factors such as hemodynamics, renin-angiotensin system and intervention of kallikrein [17, 21, 39].

Exercise Hematuria

Exercise hematuria has also been called 'stress hematuria' [8], 'athlete's kidney' [23], 'athletic pseudonephritis' [14], 'football hematuria' [22], 10000-meter hematuria' [5], etc. Hematuria may be either gross or microscopic and is present in the first and second specimens after having done an athletic event [13, 32]. The incidence of different sport events has a great variation. Sixty and 112 cases of hematuria in athletes were reported in 1980, and 1984 by Pu [30, 31], respectively, the diagnosis of 112 cases of hematuria in athletes is shown in table III. Of the 112 cases 55 cases (49.1%) were diagnosed as exercise-induced hematuria. The following clinical characteristics for exercise hematuria are summarized: (1) In trained athletes or in apparently healthy individuals, sudden appearance of hematuria after physical exercise or sports is usually related to workload. (2) The condition is most likely to occur in male runners and jumpers. (3) Except for hematuria, no special symptoms or clinical findings are found. (4) Examination of the urinary tract, blood and X-ray are normal. (5) The duration of hematuria in the majority of subjects (about 95%) is not longer than 3 days. (6) In a few subjects hematuria may recur occasionally over several years; however, the prognosis for these cases is quite good.

There may be several causes of exercise hematuria, including trauma or damage of kidney, ischemia and vasoconstriction of the renal vascular system, but the majority of reports emphasized the importance of the traumatic factor in the role of exercise hematuria, such as the concept of bladder of trauma [5, 6]. The pathogenesis of exercise hematuria is not yet clearly understood [4, 15, 19].

Exertional Hemoglobinuria

Exertional hemoglobinuria appeared to be a rather rare syndrome. Up to 1980 only about 100 cases had been reported in the literature since Fleisher described the first case in 1881 [16, 33]. We reported our first case in 1964 and 14 cases in 1974 [29]. In the last 10 years, we observed another 21 cases. With the increasing number of cases and clinical experience, we know much more about this syndrome than before, and some mistakes taken as rare occurrence were corrected. All of them were males, ranging in age from 14 to 33 years. All cases of exertional hemoglobinuria were precipitated by strenuous exercises. In 20 cases the syndrome appeared following training for long-distance running, 6 cases following training for Beijing Opera, 4 cases after training for basketball, 5 cases following marathon race, jogging and walking, and 1 case following dancing. In 23 cases (63.9%) hemoglobinuria occured in the spring season and the syndrome was closely related to specificity of the sports events with individual variation. None of them had lumbar kyposis. In 16 cases blood sugar test was negative. Three cases were complicated with hematuria and 12 cases with cylindruria.

The clinical characteristics of exertional hemoglobinuria are summarized as follows: (1) The syndrome is precipitated by exercise in the upright position, almost only in males. In the world literature only 2 cases of exertional hemoglobinuria were reported in females [9, 32, 37]. In most cases hemoglobinuria occurred following long-distance running, march and different kinds of ball games. Only 1 case has been reported following swimming [11], 1 case after bicycle exercise [40] and 1 case following karate exercise [38]. Ten cases had been reported after Japanese kendo [32]. We reported 6 cases following training for the Beijing Opera. (2) The syndrome appearing is mainly related to three factors: duration of activity, intensity of workload, and individual variability. The last seems to have the most influence. (3) Hemoglobinuria occurs more frequently following distance running on a hard surface, Davidson [12] recognized this characteristic, and therefore suggested using soft-soled shoes for prevention of the syndrome. (4) Attacks may recur after several weeks, months or years. Of 36 cases of exertional

Table IV. Urinalysis after physical training with or without use of resilient soles

Number of patients		Work bout	Urine sample					
			after exercise min	color	protein	occult blood	microscopic finding	ammonium sulfate test [7]
1	Without soles	1,200 m run	15	D	+++	+	C 0–3	+++
		1,200 m run	180	Y	±	±	C 0–1	±
	With soles	1,200 m run	15	Y	–	–	–	–
		1,200 m run	180	Y	–	–	–	–
2	Without soles	12,000 m run	15	D	++	+	WBC 1–2	+++
		16,000 m run	18	D	++	+	WBC 2–3	+++
		16,000 m run	95	D	+	+	–	+
		16,000 m run	240	Y	–	–	–	–
	With soles	12,000 m run	25	Y	±	–	WBC 0–1	–
		17,000 m run	10	Y	+	–	WBC 0–1	±
		17,000 m run	60	Y	+	–	–	–
		17,000 m run	120	Y	–	–	–	–
3	Without soles	200 m 11 run	20	D	+++	++	RBC 0–1	+++
		70 m 25 jump	60	D	++	++	RBC 0–1	+++
	With soles	200 m 11 run	25	Y	+	+	RBC 0–1	+
		70 m 25 jump	70	Y	±	–	–	±

D = Dark; Y = Yellow; C = Casts.

hemoglobinuria, follow-up observation was done in 33 cases. Thirteen cases were observed for more than 10 years. Only 2 of them continued to have attacks of hemoglobinuria after 5 years. (5) The syndrome can be prevented, diminished or avoided by the use of more resilient soles (table IV). (6) The use of large doses of vitamin C and traditional Chinese medicine for treatment have failed.

The syndrome carries all the hallmarks of acute intravascular hemolysis, which is due to the mechanical disruption of circulating red cells, but the cause of the intravascular hemolysis is not entirely clear. It has been suggested that susceptible individuals may suffer from abnormal hemolysis with ordinary activity. Davidson's [12] hypothesis is documented by several other authors. Some investigators suggested that hemoglobinuria is related to the level of haptoglobin in the body, but there is no general agreement on this point [1].

Exercise Cylindruria

The first report of exercise-induced cylindruria was made by Barach [3] just 76 years ago. He analyzed the urine of 19 marathon runners and found that 18 sediments contained both red cells and casts. Since that time, exercise cylindruria has also been reported by Amelar, Boone, Gardner, Alyea [2] and others. There are two types of casts: haline and granular casts. The finding of granular casts is more important for diagnosis. Examination of the urine sampels in distance runners and skaters showed that the incidence rate of casts increased following ultradistance exercise. The syndrome clears up rapidly, usually within 24 h. In evaluating these athletes, a prime concern is the possibility that cylindruria is due to a previously unrecognized renal disease.

Exercise Myoglobinuria

This has also been called 'acute recurrent rhabdomyolysis', 'idiopathic rhabdomyolysis', 'idiopathic myoglobinuria' etc. [18, 35]. Exercise myoglobinuria in human beings appeared to be a rare syndrome, but in recent years reports on this syndrome have been increasing. The clinical characteristics of the syndrome are intensive muscle pain and dark-brown urine after exercise, albumin in urine showing – positive test for occult blood, increase of WBC and ESR, elevation of plasma transferrin, LDH and CPK [20, 25]. The patient with exercise myoglobinuria may die due to renal failure. Knochel et al. [24] suggested that untrained subjects suffered from myoglobinuria after exhausting exercise as a result of a potassium deficit or muscle damage. Hemoglobinuria, hematuria and myoglobinuria can be observed after squat jump, and that is called 'squat jump syndrome'. Howensteine [20] reported 19 cases of this syndrome, 4 of them were cylindruria.

References

1   Allison AC, et al: The binding of hemoglobin by plasma protein (haptoglobin). Br Med J 1957; 2:1137.
2   Alyea EP: Renal response to exercise-urinary finding. JAMA 1958; 167:807.
3   Barach JG: Physiological and pathological effects of severe exercise (the marathon race) on the circulatory and renal system. Archs Intern Med 1910; 5:382.

4   Bassler TJ: Beer as prevention for runner's hematuria. Br Med J 1979; 2:1293.

5   Blacklock NJ: Bladder trauma in the long-distance runner: '10000 meters hematuria'. Br J Urol 1977; 49:129.

6   Blacklock NJ: Bladder trauma from jogging. Am Heart J 1980; 99:813.

7   Blondheim SH, et al: A simple test of myohemoglobinuria (myoglobinuria). JAMA 1958; 167:453.

8   Bruce PT: Stress hematuria. Br J Urol 1972; 49:724.

9   Buckle RM: Exertional (march)hemoglobinuria. Lancet 1965; 1:1136.

10 Castenfors J: Renal function during exercise. Acta Physiol Scand 1967; 70(suppl 293).

11 Chaiken BH, et al: Varients of march hemoglobinuria. Am J Med Sci 1953; 225:515.

12 Davidson RJL: Exertional hemoglobinuria: A report of three cases with studies on the hemolytic mechanism. J Clin Path 1964; 17:536.

13 Fred HL: Grossly bloody urine of runners. South Med J 1977; 70:1394.

14 Gardner KD: Athletic pseudonephritis, Alteration of urine sediment by athletic competition. JAMA 1956; 161:1613.

15 Gill PE, Vital DP, Tataranmi G, et al: Exercise-induced urinary abnormalities in long-distance runners. Int J Sports Med 1984; 5:237.

16 Gilligan DR, et al: March hemoglobinuria. Medicine 1941; 20:341.

17 Grimby G: Renal clearances during prolonged supine exercise at different loads. J Appl Physiol 1965; 20:1294.

18 Hamiton RW, et al: Renal function after exercise-induced myoglobinuria. Ann Intern Med 1972; 77:77.

19 Hoover DL, Cromie WJ: Theory and management of exercise-related hematuria. Phys Sportsmed 1981; 9:91.

20 Howensteine JA: Exertion-induced myoglobinuria and hemoglobinuria. JAMA 1960; 173:493.

21 Kachadorian WA, et al: Renal responses to various rates of exercise. J Appl Physiol 1970; 28:748.

22 Kishimoto T, et al: Renal hematuria resulting from exercise. Acta Urol Jap 1961; 7:896.

23 Kleiman AH: Athlete's kidney. J Urol 1960; 83:321.

24 Knochel JP, et al: The role of muscle cell injury in the pathogenesis of acute renal failure after exercise. Kidney Int 1976; 10:58.

25 Kosby MC, et al: Exercise myoglobinuria. Ann Intern Med 1972; 77:817.

26 Poortmans JR, et al: Quantitative immunological determination of twelve plasma proteins excreted in human urinae collected before and after exercise. J Clin Invest 1968; 47:386.

27 Poortmans JR, et al: Renal protein excretion after exercise in man. Med Sci Sports Exerc 1983; 15:157.

28 Poortmans JR: Exercise and renal function. Sports Med 1984; 1:125.

29 Pu Junzong, Kao Yunchiu: Exertional hemoglobinuria-analysis of 14 cases. J Beijing Med Coll 1974; 4:236.

30 Pu Junzong, Kao Yunchiu: Athlete's hematuria-Analysis of 60 cases. Chinese J Urol 1980; 1:180.

31 Pu Junzong, Kao Yunchiu: Clinical characteristics and diagnosis of hematuria in athletes-with analysis of 112 cases. Chinese J Sports Med 1984; 3:199.

32 Pu Junzong: Exercise and kidney. Chinese J Sports Med 1986; 5:103.

33 Pu Junzong, Kao Yunchiu: Exertional hemoglobinuria-analysis of 36 cases. Chinese J Sports Med 1988; 7:19.

34 Riess RW: Athletic hematuria and related phenomena. J Sports Med 1979; 19:381.

35 Rowland LP, et al: Myoglobinuria. Med Clins N Am 1972; 56:1233.

36 Siegel AJ, et al: Exercise-related hematuria. JAMA 1979; 24:397.

37 Spicer AJ: Studies on march hemoglobinuria. Br Med J 1970; 11:55.

38 Streeton JA: Traumatic hemoglobinuria caused by karate exercise. Lancet 1967; 11:191.

39 Wade CE, et al: Plasma renin activity, vasopressin and urinary excretory responses to exercise in man. J Appl Physio. 1980; 49:930.

40 Witts LT: The Paraxysmal hemoglobinuria. Lancet 1936; 11:115.

Pu Junzong, MD, Institute of Sports Medicine, Beijing Medical University, Beijing 100083 (China)

Qu Mianyu, Yu Changlong (eds): China's Sports Medicine.
Medicine Sport Sci. Basel, Karger, 1988, vol 28, pp 52–60

Anaerobic Performance of Chinese Untrained and Trained 11- to 18-Year-Old Boys and Girls

Duan Weijiang, Qiao Juxiang

Department of Exercise Physiology National Research Institute of Sports Science, Beijing, China

Introduction

It is known that energy released from anaerobic metabolism is the most important source of energy for the performance of short-duration and high-intensity exercise. Furthermore, many activities in daily life depend upon anaerobic metabolism.

There are a lot of data on aerobic capacity and power. For example, numerous studies are available on the maximal oxygen consumption of populations in different ages, from childhood to old age, and on the development of aerobic power with growth and the influence of physical activity on the aerobic working capacity. With respect to anaerobic power, although it has received attention in recent years, most reports have described methodology of its evaluation and the anaerobic performance of athletes in different events [5, 7, 10, 23, 24, 26]. Less information is available on the anaerobic characteristics of children.

In 1966 Margaria et al. [18] evaluated the energy used for short-term exercise by measuring the mechanical power output. They found that the anaerobic power increased with age and peaked at 20–30 years. Similar findings were reported by Di Prampero and Cerretelli [9] and Davies [8]. Recently, Inbar and Bar-Or [15] studied the anaerobic characteristics in Israeli male children and adolescents. They found that anaerobic power, whether expressed as absolute power values or per kg body weight, increased with age. Until now there has still been some uncertainty about the development of anaerobic performance of children and adolescents, especially of girls, who vary in their ethnic background. Thus, the purpose of the present, cross-sectional, observation is to investigate the anaerobic power of Chinese males and females aged 11–18 years, and to compare the difference in anaerobic performance between males and females and between trained and untrained youths.

Materials and Methods

Subjects

One hundred and thirty-four boys and 131 girls aged 11–18 years were randomly chosen from primary schools, high schools and university. All of them participated in the test voluntarily. The subjects were divided into four age groups: 11–12, 13–14, 15–16 and 17–18 years. Forty-seven Athletes (23 boys, 24 girls) aged 13–16 years represented the trained group. They had been trained for 1–4 years in sprint, long and high jump or middle and long distance running. Before testing, blood pressure and ECG were recorded at rest. All participants were in normal health without history of cardiopulmonary or other disease. Their physical characteristics are summarized in table I.

Measurement of Body Composition

Skinfold measurements at the triceps and subscapular sites were taken with a skinfold caliper. The mean of three measurements represented the value for each site. Considering that the Chinese and Japanese have similar physical characteristics, Nagamine's [19] equation based on sex and age was used to estimate the body density, and the percent of body fat was calculated by using Key's [17] formula.

Table I. Physical characteristics of the subjects (mean ± SD)

	Age group							
	11–12 years		13–14 years		15–16 years		17–18 years	
	M	F	M	F	M	F	M	F
N	39	37	32	38	31	25	32	31
Height, cm	147.95	148.47	163.44	157.99	168.44	158.50	172.93	160.05
	8.83	7.13	7.91	5.36	5.79	5.20	5.39	5.13
Weight, kg	38.51	35.94	48.02	45.28	55.05	49.08	59.08	50.77
	10.60	5.83	6.02	4.59	8.18	7.02	6.73	6.01
Lean body mass, kg	32.19	29.58	40.56	36.86	48.23	38.84	52.62	39.09
	6.68	3.86	5.13	2.81	4.96	4.23	5.13	3.55
Body fat, %	15.15	17.22	11.79	18.26	11.66	20.30	10.67	22.54
	6.03	4.41	2.05	5.15	6.66	5.92	4.43	6.47

Assessment of Anaerobic Power

There are several tests introduced to evaluate anaerobic power [13, 16, 21, 22, 25]. The anaerobic performance in this study was measured using the Wingate Anaerobic Test (WAnT) for legs [2, 3]. The exercise was performed on a Monark cycle ergometer. The number of pedaling revolutions was recorded continuously during 30 s. As a warm-up the subjects pedaled at a speed of 60 rpm with 0.5–1.0 kg resistance for 5 min and then tried to pedal as fast as possible for 3–5 s to familiarize themselves with the skill. After 5–10 min rest, the subjects sat on the cycle ergometer again. At the command 'start' the subject began pedaling as many revolutions as possible against a low resistance which was increased to a predetermined level within 2–3 s. At this time, a stopwatch, the electrocardiograph and the instrument for recording pedaling rate started working simultaneously. The resistance applied in this test was 0.075 kg/kg lean body mass instead of 0.075 kg/kg body weight [3]. Verbal encouragement was given throughout the 30 s test period. Two indices of the WAnT were calculated, mean power output (MP) during the 30 s (W, W/kg body weight or W/kg lean body mass) and peak power output (PP), which is the maximal power output at any 5-second period of the test (W, W/kg body weight or W/kg lean body mass).

Statistical Analysis

Comparisons of the four age groups were made using analysis of variance and the comparisons between males and females, and between trained and untrained groups were analyzed using Student-tests.

Results

Anaerobic Performance of the Males and the Females

The mean values of MP, MP/kg BW, PP and PP/kg BW of the males and the females are presented in table II. In the males, both MP and PP, whether expressed as absolute value or as the value per kg body weight, increased with growth. The differences among the four age groups were significant. In the females, the absolute values of the MP and PP also progressed significantly from 11 to 18 years of age, but for the values relative to body weight no significant differences were obtained among the four age groups.

Figure 1 presents the anaerobic performance relative to age. The values corrected for lean body mass in males still tended to increase. There were significant differences among the four age groups (p < 0.01). However, in females no such consistently increasing tendency was found.

It was observed that the increases from ages 11–12 to 13–14 in height, weight and lean body mass both in males and females accounted for more than 50% of the total increases from ages 11–12 to 17–18 years. Like the morphological variables, the progression in MP and PP between the two younger groups is also greater than between the other consecutive age groups.

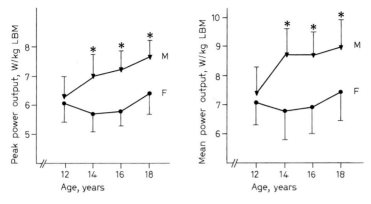

Fig. 1. Anaerobic performance per kg lean body mass (LBM) during the Wingate Anaerobic Test related to age in both sexes (mean ± 1 SD). * indicates that the males (M) had significantly higher values than the females (F) (p < 0.01).

Table II. Mean power and peak power in absolute values (W) and per kg body weight (W/kg) during the WAnT in males (M) and females (F) (mean ± SD)

Age group years	Mean power output				Peak power output			
	W		W/kg		W		W/kg	
	M	F	M	F	M	F	M	F
11–12	199.15	180.67	5.28	4.99	233.98	210.04	6.19	5.83
	42.14	33.84	0.79	0.49	54.79	41.76	0.99	0.57
13–14	283.74	213.42	6.13	4.73	352.72	251.47	7.63	5.57
	57.83	32.13	0.63	0.65	63.39	45.56	0.75	0.93
15–16	348.07	226.09	6.35	4.65	417.01	265.41	7.62	5.46
	54.37	31.08	0.68	0.56	67.50	43.37	0.98	0.90
17–18	399.61*	244.54*	6.78*	4.86	471.35*	289.49*	8.02*	5.73
	47.37	32.01	0.53	0.56	71.82	42.94	0.83	0.80

* Values significantly different among the four age groups (p < 0.01).

Compared to the males, the females had significantly lower anaerobic performance in all age groups in absolute values (p < 0.01). When expressed per body weight or lean body mass, the males still had significantly higher anaerobic power than the females. The only exception was that there was no significant difference in relative value in the group aged 11–12 between the two sexes. At 11–12 years the MP and PP of the girls were more than 90%

those of the boys. Up to the age of 17–18 the absolute values of MP and PP of the females were only about 61% those of the males, the relative values per body weight were 71% and the relative values per lean body mass were 83%.

Anaerobic Performance of the Trained and Untrained Children Aged 13–16 Years

The 15–16 and 13–14 age groups were combined as one untrained group. The physical characteristics and the anaerobic power of the trained and the untrained subjects are presented in table III. As expected, the trained groups both in males and females had significantly greater MP and PP than the untrained groups regardless of how power was expressed.

Discussion

The present results agree with previous findings [4, 15] that the anaerobic power of children and adolescents increases with age, but in our data both MP and PP in males are lower than those reported by Inbar and Bar-Or for Israeli youth. It was found by Tharp et al. [27] that in young athletes MP and PP had a high correlation with lean body mass. It is clear that the increase of anaerobic performance with growth was partly due to the increase of muscle mass with age. Some data have shown that in males from 11.5 to 17.5 years of age, the muscle mass as percentage of body weight increased from about 45.9 to 53.6% [12]. However, if MP and PP in this study were expressed relative to lean body mass, they still progressed with age in males, which is consistent with Di Prampero and Cerretelli [9]. As was pointed out by Inbar and Bar-Or [15], the age-related difference in anaerobic power, particularly among pre-pubescents, must be explained by the qualitative characteristics of the muscle.

Our data show that there were significant differences between males and females in MP and PP in absolute values. Palgi et al. [20] reported that for 10 to 14-year-old children the anaerobic power of boys was 20% higher than that of girls in absolute values but they had the same relative values. This may reflect sex differences in muscle mass and body fat. Body composition changes during growth are influenced by sex hormones. Estrogens tend to increase adipose tissue levels and have a slightly retarding effect on lean body mass, whereas androgens tend to increase lean tissue and inhibit the develop-

Table III. Physical characteristics and mean power (MP) and peak power (PP) output of the trained and untrained groups (mean ± SD)

	Male		Female	
	trained	untrained	trained	untrained
N	23	63	24	63
Age, year	14.99 0.59	15.01 0.57	15.11 0.58	15.07 0.57
Height, cm	173.70* 5.58	165.78 7.38	162.99* 4.54	158.20 5.26
Weight, kg	56.26* 5.77	50.46 8.44	47.27 5.56	46.79 5.93
LBM, kg	50.76* 5.16	44.34 6.33	40.74* 3.71	37.64 3.55
MP, W	402.77* 51.72	315.40 64.46	284.47* 45.98	218.45 32.08
MP, W/kg BW	7.16* 0.52	6.24 0.66	6.01* 0.60	4.70 0.61
MP, W/kg LBM	7.93* 0.57	7.07 0.69	6.96* 0.73	5.81 0.67
PP, W	492.02* 75.56	384.36 72.55	314.29* 56.08	257.00 44.88
PP, W/kg BW	8.71* 0.75	7.63 0.86	6.67* 0.80	5.53 0.92
PP, W/kg LBM	9.66* 0.79	8.64 0.88	7.73* 0.97	6.83 1.01

* $p < 0.01$ trained vs. untrained.

ment of body fat [6]. Previous studies have shown that in females from 13.5 through 17.5 years of age muscle mass as the percentage of body weight decreased from 45.5 to 42.5% [12]. Nevertheless, the sex difference in anaerobic performance cannot be interpreted merely by the difference in muscle mass. It was observed that even if the MP and PP were divided by lean body mass the males exhibited significantly higher MP and PP except for the group aged 11–12 years. This suggests that there must be other factors which were responsible for the sex difference in anaerobic performance. Testosterone, that has some effects on stimulating muscle glycongen production [6], may play an important role.

It was found by Grodjinovsky and Bar-Or [14] that after participating in 7 months of physical training both boys and girls revealed higher MP and PP than the control groups, while the results obtained by Armstrong et al. [1] indicated that trained boys displayed greater anaerobic performance in absolute values than untrained ones but there were no significant differences in the values relative to body weight. As we can see in table III, the height, weight and lean body mass in males, and the height and lean body mass in females of the trained groups were significantly higher than those of the untrained groups. Therefore, it is possible that the higher anaerobic performance in the trained groups was due to their large body size, but for the values relative to the lean body mass the trained groups still showed greater anaerobic power. This must be explained by the high concentration of CP and ATP in trained muscles and the increase of phosphofructokinase after training [11]. The present data led us to believe that physical training has some effects on improvement of anaerobic performance during growth. However, our results were just from a cross-sectional study. Further longitudinal study should be done to identify the effects of physical training on the development of anaerobic capacity. For instance, to what extent can physical training increase the anaerobic capacity and how can the various kinds of training programs, endurance, strength and sprint training, influence the development of anaerobic performance.

In conclusion, the development of anaerobic power of children and adolescents has its own characteristics. The anaerobic performance of Chinese females was significantly inferior to that of males after 13 years of age, regardless of how it was expressed. During 11–12 years of age there were significant differences in absolute values between the two sexes but no significant differences were found in the values relative to body weight and lean body mass. This is due to the fact that males have more muscle mass and less body fat than females. Testosterone may play some role in the differences of anaerobic power related to sex and, perhaps, age. Physical training may improve anaerobic performance during growth.

Summary

To investigate the anaerobic power of children and adolescents during growth, 265 untrained males and females aged 11–18 years and 47 trained males and females aged 13–16 years were tested using the Wingate Anaerobic Test. The males in the present test had a lower anaerobic power output than Israeli youths both in absolute values and values relative to body weight. Compared to the males, the females showed significantly lower anaerobic power output whether expressed in absolute values, values per kg body weight or values per kg lean body mass. However, between males and females of 11–12 years of age, there were no significant differences when the values were expressed per body weight and per lean body mass. The trained groups in both sexes had a significantly higher anaerobic performance than the age-matched untrained groups. The data suggest that the development of anaerobic performance in children has its own characteristics and was related to the growth of body size, but the differences related to age and sex cannot be explained only by the body size or by lean body mass.

References

1   Armstrong N, Davies B, Heal M: The specificity of energy utilisation by trained and untrained adolescent boys. Br J Sports Med 1983; 17:193–199.

2   Bar-Or O, Dotan R, Inbar O: A 30 second all-out ergometric test; its reliability and validity (abstract). Isr J Med Sci 1977; 13:326.

3   Bar-Or O: The Wingate anaerobic test, characteristics and applications. Symbioses 1981; 13:157–172.

4   Bar-Or O: The growth and development of children's physiologic and perceptional responses to exercise. 8th Congr Paediatric Work Physiology, Joutsa 1981. Children and Sports, ed. 1. Paediatric Work Physiology. Berlin, Springer, 1984, pp 3–17.

5   Bhanot JL, Sidhu LS: Maximal anaerobic power in Indian national hockey players. Br J Sports Med 1983; 17:34–39.

6   Brooks GA, Fahey TD: Exercise physiology, ed 1. New York, Wiley, 1984, pp 638–646.

7   Crielaard, JM, Pirnay F: Anaerobic and aerobic power of top athletes. Eur J Appl Physiol 1981; 47:295–300.

8   Davies CTM: Human power output in exercise of short duration in relation to body size and composition. Ergonomics 1969; 14:245–256.

9   Di Prampero PE, Cerretelli P: Maximal muscular power (aerobic and anaerobic) in African natives. Ergonomics 1969; 12:51–59.

10 Di Prampero PE, Limas FP, Sassi G: Maximal muscular power aerobic and anaerobic, in 116 athletes performing at the XIXth Olympic Games in Mexico. Ergonomics 1970; 13:665–674.

11 Eriksson BO, Gollnick PD, Saltin B: Muscle metabolism and enzyme activities after training in boys 11–13 years old. Acta Physiol Scand 1973; 87:485:497.

12 Falkner F, Tanner JM: Human growth, ed 1. New York, Plenum Press, 1978, p 283.

13 Fox EL: Measurement of the maximal alactic (phosphagen) capacity in man. Med Sci Sports 1973; 5:66.

14 Grodjinovsky A, Bar-Or O: Influence of added physical education hours upon anaerobic capacity, adiposity, and grip strength in 12 to 13 year old children enrolled in a sports class. 8th Congr Paediatric Work Physiology, Joutsa 1981. Children and Sport, ed 1. Berlin, Springer, 1984, pp 162–169.

15 Inbar O, Bar-Or O: Anaerobic characteristics in male children and adolescents. Med Sci Sports Exer 1986; 18:264–269.

16 Katch V, Weltman A, Martin R, et al: Optimal test characteristics for maximal anaerobic work in the bicycle ergometer. Res Qu 1977; 48:319–327.

17 Key A: Body fat in adult man. Physiol Ref 1953; 33:245.

18   Margaria R, Aghemo P, Rovelli E: Measurement of muscular power (anaerobic) in man. J Appl Physiol 1966; 21:1662–1664.

19   Nagamine S: Estimate body fat by skinfold. J Jap Ass Med 1972; 68:919.

20   Palgi Y, Gutin B, Young J, et al: Physiologic and anthropometric factors underlying endurance performance in children. Int J Sports Med 1984; 5:67–73.

21   Sargeant AJ: Measurement of maximal short-term (anaerobic) power out-put in man. J Physiol 1980; 307:12–13.

22   Sawaka MN, Tahamont MV, Fitzgerald PI, et al: Alactic capacity and power: reliability and interpretation. Eur J Appl Physiol 1980; 45:109–116.

23   Schnabel A, Kindermann W: Assessment of anaerobic capacity in runners. Eur J Appl Physiol 1983; 52:42–46.

24   Sidhu LS: Maximal anaerobic power in national level Indian players. Br J Sports Med 1981; 15:265–268.

25   Simoneau JA, Lortie G, Boulay MR, et al: Test of anaerobic alactacid and lactacid capacities; description and reliability. Can J Appl Spt Sci 1983; 8:266–270.

26   Taunton JE, Maron H, Wilkinson JG: Anaerobic performance in middle and long distance runners. Can J Appl Spt Sci 1981; 6:109–113.

27   Tharp GD, Johnson GO, Thorland WG: Measurement of anaerobic power and capacity in elite young track athletes using the Wingate test. J Sports Med Phys Fitness 1984; 24:100–106.

Duan Weijiang, MD, Department of Exercise Physiology, National Research Institute of Sports Science, 11 Tiyuguan Road, Beijing 100061 (China)

Qu Mianyu, Yu Changlong (eds): China's Sports Medicine.
Medicine Sport Sci. Basel, Karger, 1988, vol 28, pp 61–69

Functional Training after Reconstruction of the Thumb through Free Transplantation of the Second Toe

Fan Zhenhua, Chen Xiner, Tu Danyun

Department of Sports Medicine, Hua-Shan Hospital, Shanghai Medical University, Shanghai, China

Free transplantation of the second toe is the most favorable procedure to reconstruct a lost thumb. It provides ideal restoration of the internal structure as well as the outward appearance of the thumb and thus allows satisfactory functional recovery [1].

Disuse atrophy of the thumb muscles always follows thumb amputation. Surgical trauma and fixation after surgery aggravate the muscle atrophy and give rise to joint contracture and tissue adhesion. All of these result in functional limitation of the replantated thumb in various degrees of severity requiring to be resolved with a special program of functional training. This paper is aimed to introduce an approach of functional training and its results.

Basic Condition of Cases

This group of patients consists of 39 cases including 26 males and 13 females. The age distribution was 18–19: 2 cases; 20–29: 26 cases; 30–39: 7 cases; 40 and above: 4 cases. Twenty-two cases lost their right thumb while 17 cases their left. In 19 cases, thumb amputations were complicated with injuries of other parts of the hands. The causes of the traumata were mainly industrial injuries.

Functional training began immediately after the removal of external and internal fixations. It is about 4 and 8 weeks after surgery in cases with joint capsule sutured and cases with bone inlaid, respectively.

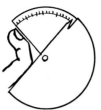

Fig. 1. Measurement of thumb flexion.

Functional Evaluation

The following functional tests were carried out before the training program and were repeated after each 10 training sessions.

Range of Motion (ROM) Measurement
Flexion and Extention Range of the Thumb. A finger angurometer was used to measure flexion and extention range of metacarpo-phalangeal and interphalangeal joints. Data from active and passive motion were documented separately if there was significant difference between the two readings. In the reconstructed thumb two interphalangeal joints exist, i.e. proximal and distal which were taken for one joint when measured, i.e. the angle between the proximal and distal segment of the thumb was documented (fig. 1).

Abduction of the Thumb. Put the carpo-metacarpal joint of the thumb at 45 degrees flexion and record the maximal distance between the points of the radial end of the metacarpal line and the ulnar end of the proximal interphalangeal line.

Opposition. Thumb opposition function was marked as '1', '2', '3', '4' and '5', respectively, when the thumb could touch the top of the 2nd, 3rd, 4th, 5th finger and the root of the 5th finger. Care should be taken not to substitute opposition with thumb adduction and flexion.

Muscle Strength
Grip and pinch strength were measured with a gripmeter.

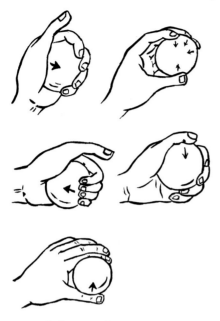

Fig. 2. Ball compression.

Method

All the patients received basal functional training in hospital every day or every other day and were encouraged to do self-care, housework, and to manipulate some kind of tools at home.

Basal functional training including:

Warm-up: Make a fist and extend the fingers alternatively 10 times, then abduct and adduct the fingers 10 times.

Strengthening exercises: All extrinsic and intrinsic muscles of the thumb as well as other fingers can be strengthened through the following exercise: Compress a rubber ball or a roll of sponge to strengthen the flexors, adductor and oppositor of the thumb and the flexors of other fingers (fig. 2).

Rubber band pulling: Pull the rubber bands fixed on a wooden frame to strengthen the extensors, adductors and abductors of the thumb and other fingers (fig. 3).

According to the general rule of muscle strengthening exercise, great resistance with limited repetition favors muscle strength, while moderate resistance with great repetition favors muscle endurance [2]. Patients were advised to do each of the above exercises with maximal effort so as to obtain obvious feeling of local muscle fatigue within 10 repetitions and repeat this course 2–3 times after short breaks.

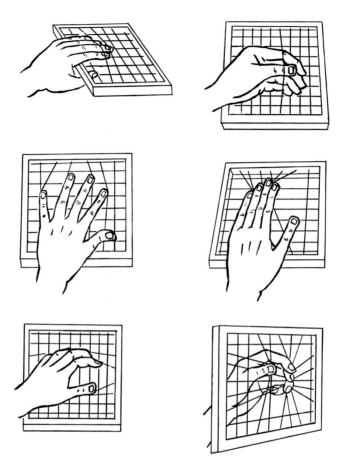

Fig. 3. Pulling rubber bands with wooden frame.

Strengthening exercise sessions were carried out once daily or every other day to allow sufficient intervals for muscle recovery and over-recovery to take place, as it is generally believed that over-recovery from muscle fatigue is the basis for muscle volume and strength increase.

ROM Exercises

The main causes of ROM limitation are contracture of fibrous tissues including joint capsule, ligaments, tendons and adhesion formation. Stretching the fibrous tissues with active and passive movement is the general approach to improve ROM. The fibrous tissues, according to their mechanical property, show great resistance to sudden and strong stretching but can be

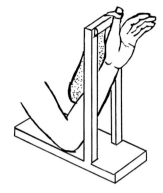
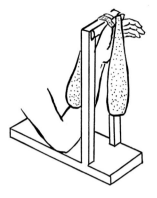

Fig. 4. Flexion traction of the thumb.   *Fig. 5.* Extension traction of the thumb.

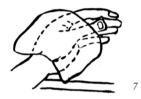

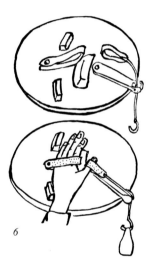
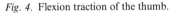

Fig. 6. Abduction traction of the thumb.
Fig. 7. Opposition traction of the thumb.

elongated more easily under moderate and sustained stretching [3]. So an intermittent angular traction program [4] was adopted to restore ROM of the thumb. In this procedure, the proximal segment of the joint to be treated was fixed on a special brace or instrument, then the distal segment was tractioned along a selected direction with a weight that caused moderate pain at the joint but could be tolerated easily by the patients (fig. 4–7). Traction was sustained for 10–15 min at a time and was done 3–4 times a day if feasible.

Patients were advised to press the joints against desired directions steadily for 5–10 min at a time and several times a day to accelerate the improvement of ROM (fig. 8). This procedure is better done in conjunction with hot immersion.

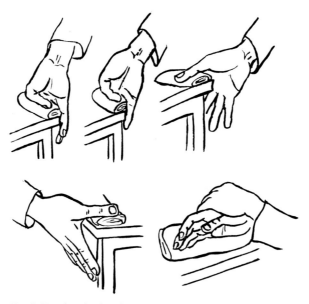

Fig. 8. Pressing the thumb joints against desired directions.

Results

This group of 39 cases was treated on average for 49.4 sessions (18–29 sessions: 25 cases; 40–59 sessions: 7 cases; 60–69 sessions: 3 cases; more than 100 sessions: 4 cases).

Tables I and II show the ROM of the reconstructed thumb before and after the training program. All data except extension of the inter-phalangeal joint showed significant improvement.

Table III shows the strength of the hand. The readings were doubled after training and reached 49–80% of that of the uninjured side.

The improvement of most functional variables was fast at the first 10 sessions of exercise and then slowed down during the whole course of the training program.

The overall basal function of the thumb was evaluated according to the scale shown in table IV. The results of the evaluation are shown in table V. The rate of 'good' and 'excellent' was about 28% before training and reached 87% after training.

Well recovery of hand function does not require full recovery of ROM and strength of the hand. For example, in 2 male cases in this series with the thumb of the dominant hand reconstructed, the recovery of flexion of the

Table I. ROM of the thumb

	Uninjured side	Injured side				
		before training	%	after training	%	p
Metacarpophalangeal						
Flexion	65.56 ± 1.54	30.58 ± 1.98	47[1]	45.29 ± 2.14	69	< 0.001
Extension	> 180	164.26 ± 1.56	86[2]	174.48 ± 1.62	95	< 0.001
Interphalangeal						
Flexion	82.68 ± 1.16	35.83 ± 3.22	43[1]	56.28 ± 3.35	68	< 0.001
Extension	> 180	156.78 ± 2.35	76[2]	153.81 ± 2.58	73	> 0.1
Thumb abduction cm						
Male	5.18 ± 0.16	3.76 ± 0.27	71[1]	4.47 ± 0.25	86	< 0.001
Female	4.33 ± 0.12	2.33 ± 0.26	54[1]	3.26 ± 0.29	75	< 0.001

[1] Take uninjured side as 100 %.
[2] Take 180-injured side as 100 %.

Table II. Case distribution in opposition function

	Functional scale						
	0	1	2	3	4	5	total
Before training	2	1	4	7	10	0	24
After training	1	0	1	2	12	8	24

$x^2 = 8.89$, $p < 0.005$.

Table III. Strength of the hands

	Uninjured side	Injured side				
		before training	%	after training	%	p
Grip						
Male	36.78 ± 1.31	13.88 ± 1.85	38	29.53 ± 1.76	80	< 0.001
Female	25.38 ± 1.63	7.70 ± 1.31	30	14.75 ± 2.74	58	< 0.025
Pinch						
Male	11.84 ± 0.57	3.18 ± 0.50	29	6.67 ± 0.56	56	< 0.001
Female	9.11 ± 0.50	2.46 ± 0.46	27	4.46 ± 0.42	49	< 0.005

Table IV. Scale of functional evaluation

	Points gained			
	1	2	3	4
Metacarpophalangeal joint				
Flexion	0–14	15–29	30–44	45–
Extension	0–14	15–29	30–44	45–
Interphalangeal Joint				
Flexion	0–19	20–39	40–59	60–
Extension	0–19	20–39	40–59	60–
Thumb abduction				
Male	0–1.9	2–2.9	3–3.9	4–
Female	0–0.9	1–1.9	2–2.9	3–
Grip power				
Male	0–8	9–17	18–26	27–
Female	0–5	6–11	12–17	18–
Pinch power				
Male	0–2.5	3–5.5	6–8.5	9–
Female	0–2.5	3–4.5	5–6.5	7–
Opposition	1	2	3	4

Table V. Result of functional evaluation

	Total points gain	Cases	
		before training	after training
Very poor	≤ 13	0	0
Poor	14–20	28	5
Good	21–27	11	32
Excellent	28	0	2

$x^2 = 27.79$, $p < 0.0015$.

metacarpo-phalangeal joint and extension of the interphalangeal joint were about 60 and 56%, pinch power were 47 and 44%, opposition functions were '4' and '3'. Both of the cases could perform self-care such as dressing and cleaning; could write and use chopsticks freely, they could also manipulate tools including hammer, clamp, screw-driver and spanner, and returned to their original job (technician and machine mender). Other examples were 3 female cases with recovery in ROM and strength resembling the 2 cases mentioned above. They could do fine work such as manual weaving, sewing and embroidery with the reconstructed thumb. It seems that practical hand function can be satisfactorily restored when the basal function (i.e. ROM and strength) of the hand reaches the 'good' grade.

Discussion

The complex and fine functional motion of the hand is based mainly on ROM and strength of all fingers, especially the thumb. So, as the ROM and strength of the reconstructed thumb is improved to a considerable degree through ROM and strength exercise, the practical hand function can be restored without difficulty.

It has been proved effective to use a set of simple wooden apparatus in ROM and strength exercise of the reconstructed thumb. We can stretch the distal joint through active, passive motion and sustained traction to pull the adhered tendon to glide distally, but only active contraction of the muscle can pull the tendon to glide proximally. In many cases, active muscle contraction is not sufficient to loosen an adhered tendon. In 8 cases of this series, the average range of interphalangeal joint flexion reached in active motion was 27.5 degrees less than that in passive motion, and in 6 cases the difference between active and passive extension of this joint was 35.7 degrees. These phenomena show delay in the recovery of active motion due to tendon adhesion. Surgical intervention was applied to 2 cases of this series as the active ROM did not recover to a suitable degree.

Summary

An approach to functional training using a set of simple wooden apparatus after reconstruction of the thumb through free transplantation of the second toe was introduced and the satisfactory results gained in a series of 39 cases was reported. It showed that practical function of the hand can be restored on the basis of improved ROM and strength of the reconstructed thumb. Surgical release of the adhered tendon was indicated in a few cases while the recovery of active ROM of the thumb was significantly delayed to passive ROM.

References

1   Yang Dongyue: Thumb reconstruction through free transplantation of the second toe, a report of 40 cases. Chin J Surg 1977; 15:13.
2   Rusk HA: Principles of therapeutic exercise and muscle re-education; in Rehabilitation Medicine, ed 2, p 99. St Louis, Mosby, 1964.
3   Kottke FJ, et al: The rationale for prolonged stretching for correction of shortening of connective tissue. Arch Phys Med 1966; 47:345.
4   Fan Zhenhua, Tu Danyun: Use intermittent traction to improve articular mobility. A report of 1424 cases. All-China Academic Discussion About Sports Sciences, 1980.

Fan Zhenhua, MD, Department of Sports Medicine, Hua-Shan Hospital, Shanghai Medical University, Shanghai 200040 (China)

Qu Mianyu, Yu Changlong (eds): China's Sports Medicine.
Medicine Sport Sci. Basel, Karger, 1988, vol 28, pp 70–80

Physiological Studies of Tai Ji Quan in China

Xu Shengwen, Fan Zhenhua

Department of Sports Medicine, Hua-Shan Hospital, Shanghai Medical University,
Shanghai, China

Tai Ji Quan is a representative of Chinese traditional conditioning exercise. It consists of a series of motions which are gentle and smooth, complex and harmonic, and relaxing and fluent. It combines muscle exercise with breath and mind regulation. Its aim is to reach mental calm through body motion. All of these characteristics make Tai Ji Quan significantly different from most other exercises. Moreover, Tai Ji Quan especially suits the aged and patients with chronic diseases because of its moderate intensity, steady rhythm, and hence low physical and mental tension produced. Tai Ji Quan has its special position in rehabilitation medicine and has been introduced to more and more countries besides China.

In China, medical and physiological studies about Tai Ji Quan began in the late 1950s. This paper is aimed to review the main achievements gained so far as recorded in the literature.

Studies on Chronic Effects of Tai Ji Quan

Anthropometric Studies

In 1959, the Institute of Sports Medicine of Beijing Medical College made a comprehensive medical study including an anthropometric study for 31 aged men who had been practising Tai Ji Quan regularly for 40 years on average [1]. Higher readings were gained in most items from the aged Tai Ji Quan group in comparison with the control group, especially in items such as difference of thoracic circumference at inhalation and exhalation, vital capacity and grip power. Limb circumferences and skin fold thickness were

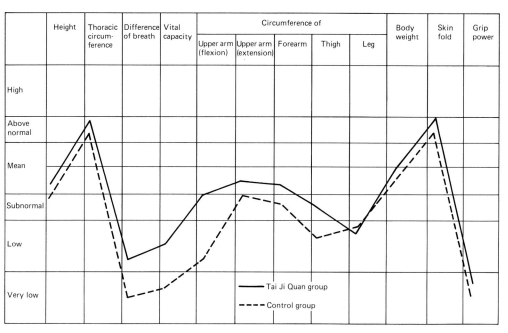

Fig. 1. Body figure of aged Tai Ji Quan players.

comparable to or higher than that of a young control group. Figure 1 shows an example of the body figure developed from this study.

In 1964, Fan Zhenhua et al. [2] obtained a similar result in a study on 80 aged men who had been practising Tai Ji Quan for an average of 25 years.

Liang Yonghai et al. [3] found that the overweight which occurred in 32 aged Tai Ji Quan players was much less than in the control group (13.8%:26%). The sex and age distributions were not carefully balanced in the two groups in this study.

All of these materials suggest a favorable effect of Tai Ji Quan in retarding dystrophic changes associated with aging.

Bones and Joints

A detailed clinical and roentgenologic study was made at the Institute of Sports Medicine of Beijing Medical College [1]. In 31 aged Tai Ji Quan players, the incidence of malalignment of the spine was much lower than in the control group (25.8%:47.2%). The incidences of round back were 13 and 28% in the two groups.

Table I. Percent of cases that can reach the floor with finger tip when bending

Source of material	Tai Ji Quan group	Control group
Beijing [1]	85.7	20.7
Shanhai [2]	87.2	15.6
Kwangchow [3]	65.8	40.0

Table II. Incidence of roentgenologic changes

	Tai Ji Quan group	Control group
Osteoporosis	36.6	63.8
Fish vertebrae	3.3	19.4
Vertebral body compression	6.6	30.5

Table III. Incidence of vertebral lip formation (%)

Age years	Tai Ji Quan group		Control group	
	total	III	total	III
50–59	17.9	0	22.9	14
60–69	40.3	20	36.4	8
70–79	39.6	0	62.0	20
80–89	56.7	0	57.8	27

Three studies [1, 3] found that the flexibility of the spine was much better in aged Tai Ji Quan players than in the control groups (table I), suggesting less degenerative changes in the lumbar vertebrae and their subsidiary structures and better elasticity in the spinal muscles and ligments as a result of playing Tai Ji Quan.

Roentgenologic study of the lumbar spine[1] showed a lower incidence of osteoporosis, fish vertebrae and vertebral body compression (table II) and fewer vertebrae involved.

In the Tai Ji Quan group, the incidence and degree of lip formation of the lumbar vertebrae were both lower and did not reach the third degree in general, while in the control group, more bone bridges formed (table III).

From the above findings, Tai Ji Quan playing is thought to be beneficial to delay degenerative changes of the spine with aging and to reduce chronic low back pain.

Cardiovascular System

Exercise tests for cardiovascular function were made on 32 aged Tai Ji Quan players at the Institute of Sports Medicine of Beijing Medical College [1]. All subjects were advised to climb up and down a step of 40 cm in height 15 times a minute. All Tai Ji Quan players except one finished this designed exercise without difficulty, while in the control group, the percentage of cases who completed the exercise task was reduced with aging: 85.9, 54.5, 25.0 and 0% in the groups aged 50–59, 60–69, 70–79 and 80–89 years, respectively. In the Tai Ji Quan group, no abnormal reaction pattern was found except for hypertensive reaction (excessive rise of SBP and HR with a rise of DBP after exercise) in 5 cases. While in the control group, there were pathological reactions such as a ladder-shaped rise of the SBP (SBP rises step by step after designed exercise) and a feeble reaction (excessive rise of HR with inadequate rise of SBP) each seen in 4 cases, suggesting a deterioration of myocardial reserve.

The percentage of undesirable ECG reactions, including elongation of P-R, QRS or QT intervals, reduced RV5 range, depression of ST more than 0.5 mm and reversed T wave, was 28.2% in the Tai Ji Quan group but reached 41.3% in the control group.

The testing exercise used by Liang Yonghai et al. [3] was squatting down and standing up 20 times. Compared with the control group, they found that the HR of the Tai Ji Quan group recovered faster after exercise and showed a higher SBP/HR rate. The differences were statistically significant.

Average blood pressure of the aged Tai Ji Quan group reported by the Institute of Sports Medicine of Beijing Medical College [1] was 134.1/80.8 mm Hg. The SBP was lower by 20 mm Hg than that of the control group. Roentgenological measurement of the heart area showed no significant difference between the two groups. Average blood pressure of 80 aged Tai Ji Quan players evaluated in Shanghai [2] was 134.4/74.6 mm Hg. It did not differ from the 143.6/76.1 mm Hg of the control group. But ¼ of the control group members were taking or had been taking antihypertensive drugs, while in the Tai Ji Quan group, none acknowledged such drug taking.

A study of cardiac function using the B-type echocardiogram by Zhang Wenli et al. [4] showed an enlarged left ventricle and increased cardiac output and systolic volume in Tai Ji Quan players. No significant difference was found between Chen-style and Yang-style Tai Ji Quan players.

Recently, Cai Shijue et al. [5] reported an observation on the stability of the automatic nervous system in cardiovascular regulation. After immersion of both hands in 4 °C water for 1 min, no significant change in BP was found

Table IV. Comparison of respiratory functions

	Tai Ji Quan group	Control group	Value
% of VC to predicted VC	88.5	88.3	>0.05
% of maximum ventilation to predicted maximum ventilation	106.0	90.4	< 0.05
First-second VC	69.5	65.2	< 0.05
% of ventilation reserve	91.2	85.3	< 0.01
% of residue volume to VC	38.3	40.3	> 0.05
CO absorption rate	51.7	45.5	< 0.01
pCO_2, mm Hg	43.9	46.7	< 0.01
Gas distribution, % N_2 difference	3.9	4.4	> 0.05
Range of diaphragm motion, cm	6.8	4.5	< 0.01

in the Tai Ji Quan players, while in the control group, an obvious rise in BP was noted.

According to these studies, Tai Ji Quan was believed to be effective in improving cardiovascular function and preventing hypertension.

Respiratory System

In a study by the Institute of Sports Medicine of Beijing Medical College [1], an aged Tai Ji Quan group was superior to a control group in average vital capacity (2,743 vs. 2,451 ml) and the average difference between chest circumferences at inspiration and at expiration (4.3 vs. 3.8 cm).

Xu Shengwen et al. [6] made a study of respiratory function in 36 aged Tai Ji Quan teachers. The results are summarized in table IV. It is worthwhile noting that the indices of Tai Ji Quan teachers referring to ventilation and diffusion function were obviously superior to that of the control group, while the indices mainly referring to lung structure, the difference between the two groups was not obvious.

Blood Lipid Levels

To determine the influence of Tai Ji Quan on blood lipid levels, Jiang Jianxin [7] observed a series of 32 patients admitted for various diseases. The subjects were divided into a Tai Ji Quan group (15 cases) and a control group (17 cases). Members of the Tai Ji Quan group practised Tai Ji Quan for 40 min daily. Changes in the blood lipid levels after 1 month are shown in table V.

In the Tai Ji Quan group, there was a significant rise in the anti-atherosclerosis index (HDL-C/TC) and a lowering in the cause-atherosclerosis

Table V. Changes in blood lipid levels

	Tai Ji Quan group	Control group
TG	–	–
TC	–	↓
HDL-C	↑	↓
LDL-C	–	–
HDL-C/TC	↑	–
TC-HDL-C/HDL-C	↓	–

Table VI. A comparison of the three groups in serum endocrine levels

Items	A Tai Ji group 51	B control group 1 47	C control group 2 15	A:B	B:C	A:C
F, ng/dl	14.74 ± 4.73	15.23 ± 7.67	14.20 ± 3.92	> 0.05	> 0.05	> 0.05
TSH, μU/ml	4.80 ± 3.05	3.80 ± 1.55	3.10 ± 1.15	< 0.05	> 0.05	< 0.05
T$_3$, ng/ml	0.93 ± 0.20	0.84 ± 0.21	1.51 ± 0.31	< 0.05	< 0.01	< 0.05
T$_4$, ng/ml	69.97 ± 23.87	73.60 ± 31.96	104.97 ± 38.60	> 0.05	< 0.05	< 0.01
rT$_3$, ng/ml	30.26 ± 7.77	28.79 ± 4.96	37.22 ± 7.64	> 0.05	< 0.01	< 0.01
FSH, mIU/ml	16.54 ± 15.16	11.05 ± 6.08	4.85 ± 1.58	< 0.05	< 0.01	< 0.01
LH, mIU/ml	11.74 ± 13.19	8.03 ± 5.95	4.41 ± 1.31	> 0.05	< 0.01	< 0.05
T, ng/dl	680.00 ± 430.00[a]	510.00 ± 151.00	679.00 ± 173.00[b]	< 0.05	< 0.01	> 0.05
E$_2$, pg/ml	63.91 ± 17.14	54.74 ± 18.62[c]	50.70 ± 7.14[d]	< 0.05	> 0.05	< 0.05
PRL, ng/ml	7.06 ± 3.46	6.34 ± 2.75	8.25 ± 3.21	> 0.05	> 0.05	> 0.05

group 1 = Aged; group 2 = adult, [a]n = 50; [b]n = 12; [c]n = 46; [d]n = 10.

index (TC-HDL-C/HDL-C). Both of the two indices were not changed in the control group. The author pointed out that lowering of the TC level is not always beneficial to health, the rise of the HDL-C level is of more importance. This study suggests that to improve the blood lipid level, it is not required to do exercise of higher intensity than considered before.

Serum Endocrine Levels

Xu Shengwen and Wang Wenjian [8] made observations on the neuroendocrine function of the inferior colliculus, pituitary gland and gonad axis on an aged Tai Ji Quan group (group A, 51 cases), an aged control group (group B, 47 cases), and an adult control group (group C, 17 cases). A comparison of serum endocrine levels is shown in table VI.

In analyzing the material shown in table VI, the authors pointed out that the level of target endocrines including T3, T4, rT3 and T decreases with aging. The level of pituitary-stimulating hormones such as TSH, FSH and LH increases with aging. It may be looked upon as a functional compensation of the pituitary gland. However, this compensation is not complete as the target endocrine levels remain lower in the two aged groups than in the adult control group. An obvious difference of TSH and FSH found between the two aged groups shows a stronger compensation action of putuitary gland in the Tai Ji Quan group than in the aged control group. Moreover, a higher level of T3 in the Tai Ji Quan group may be of significance in keeping normal metabolism and retarding the aging process.

Immunity Function

The rosette-forming procedure was used by Sun Xusheng et al. [9] to explore the influence of Tai Ji Quan on cell immunity function with an aged Tai Ji Quan group and a control group consisting of 30 cases each. The total rosettes formed (Et) and active rosette (Ea) number in the Tai Ji Quan group were both superior to that of the control group ($p < 0.01$) (table VII). Immediately after Tai Ji Quan exercise, Et and Ea of the Tai Ji Quan group were both raised. According to these findings, the author proposed a favorable effect of Tai Ji Quan on nonspecific cell immunity.

'Shen' Deficiency

'Shen' deficiency is a special term of Chinese traditional medicine. It consists of a series of symptoms in accordance with appearances associated with aging. A points counting method of 'Shen' deficiency diagnosis was used by Fan Zhenhua et al. [2] for 80 aged Tai Ji Quan players. The incidence of 'Shen' deficiency was found to be 18%, corresponding to $\frac{1}{3}$ of that of the control group. This finding may be meaningful when considered together with the changes of endocrine function mentioned above.

Immediate Physiological Changes during Tai Ji Quan Exercise

Energy Consumption

Data about the immediate physiological changes gained by several authors may be summarized roughly and are shown in table VIII.

Although different units were used by authors, a rough comparison of the energy cost can be made among Tai Ji Quan of different styles. The

Table VII. Number of rosettes formed

	Et	Ea
At rest		
Tai Ji Quan group	1,449 + 86	685 + 42
Control group	713 + 48	287 + 22
Rosette formation increased after Tai Ji Quan exercise	1,315 + 156	1,224 + 110

Table VIII. Immediate physiological changes

Author	Group size	Style of Tai Ji Quan	Physiological changes				Energy cost
			HR	BP	R	venti-lation	
Huang Shijun et al., [10]	20	simplified	105	128/71	21.8	8.54	2.3 cal/min
Zhuo Dahong [11]	11	Yang style	131	146/86	23.2	24.6	4,1 met
Zhang Wenli et al. [4]	14	Chen style	135				2.76 cal/m²·min
	13	Yang style	118				1.76 cal/m²·min
Chao Wenyuan [12]	10	?	107			15.9	3 met

Table IX. Energy cost of Tai Ji Quan with high and low postures

Style	Energy cost, cal/m²·min			duration min
	high posture	low posture	p	
Chen	2.70	4.27	< 0.01	6
Yang	1.04	1.77	< 0.01	17
Simplified	1.24	1.91	< 0.01	5

highest reading seen in Chen style Tai Ji Quan corresponds to the energy cost when walking at a normal pace. The energy cost during the Yang style and simplified style were even lower.

Chen Wenhe and Chao Fusheng [13] compared the energy consumption when high posture and low posture (with knee joints kept at about 30 and 60° flexion, respectively) were adopted in Tai Ji Quan exercise (table IX).

Yang style Tai Ji Quan showed a lower energy cost than Chen style, but due to its longer duration, the total energy consumption corresponded to the

Chen style. There was significant difference of energy cost when high and low postures were adopted. The highest one can be fourfold of the lowest one, indicating a considerable range of exercise intensity for option.

Chao Wenyuan [12] found a significant higher energy cost in high level Tai Ji Quan players than in general players during Tai Ji Quan exercise of the same style, suggesting stronger internal physiological changes that occurred in excellent Tai Ji Quan players and thus a better conditioning effect may be reached.

Electroencephalographic Study

In a study on 17 aged Tai Ji Quan players and 12 control aged men, Ju Zhiping et al. [14] found no significant difference at rest EEG between the two groups. When the aged Tai Ji Quan players were ordered to imagine Tai Ji Quan exercise, a prolonged alpha-rhythm with increasing height was seen in the anterior area of both hemispheres. These phenomena resembled somewhat EEG changes seen during Chi-Gong practise.

Hu Huaizhong et al. [15] examined EEG changes on 10 excellent Tai Ji Quan players during imaginary Tai Ji Quan exercise. A general increase in alpha-rhythm frequency was seen in 7 cases. Power of main frequency decreased. Instead of alpha-rhythm, there was a rise of a series of low and fast waves indicating de-synchronism of the alpha-rhythm. Afterwards, synchronism and de-synchronism of the alpha-rhythm appeared alternatively. The author suggested that EEG changes during imaginary Tai Ji Quan exercise have their own characteristics, differing from those seen during Chi-Gong practising and sleep. De-synchronism and synchronism reflect enhancement of exciting and inhibition processes, respectively. Changes of de-synchronism and synchronism in sequence during imaginary Tai Ji Quan exercise indicated an alternative appearance of a different functional complex which was believed to be beneficial to intellectual activity.

Summary

A series of researches on the physiological effects of Tai Ji Quan carried out in China was reviewed in this paper. The intensity of Tai Ji Quan of different style and posture was established in general. The effect of Tai Ji Quan in delaying body dystrophy and structural and functional changes of the spine associated with aging were explored in some detail. Some virtues of Tai Ji Quan players in cardiovascular and respiratory function as well as blood lipid levels were expounded. Studies about the effects of Tai Ji Quan on endocrine levels and immune function have also been started and some interesting results have been obtained. The research work is rather extensive in area but remains to be explored further, and some findings remain to be confirmed.

As mentioned at the beginning of this paper, Tai Ji Quan as an item of conditioning and therapeutic exercise, has its outstanding characteristics which may give rise to some special physiological effects. EEG changes during imaginary Tai Ji Quan exercise and the higher energy consumption documented during Tai Ji Quan exercise of high level Tai Ji Quan players revealed some interesting phenomena. It may be of great value to carry out further studies in this direction.

References

1   Institute of Sports Medicine of Beijing Medical College: A medical observation on aged Tai Ji Quan players. J Beijing Med Coll 1959; 1:73.

2   Fan Zhenhua, et al: A primary research of the effect of Tai Ji Quan on health improving and longevity. Selected collection of 1964's all China Academic Discussion about Sports Science, Division of Sports Physiology and Sports Medicine, part II, p 180. People's Publishing House of Physical Culture, 1966.

3   Liang Yonghai, et al: A summary of medical evaluation on 120 aged Tai Ji Quan players. Materials of Sports Science, Division of Sports Medicine, vol 6, p 27. Institute of Sports Science, Kwandong, 1980.

4   Zhang Wenli, et al: The physiological observation of Tai Ji-Quan, in Beijing International Conference on Sports Medicine (abstracts of papers). Chinese Association of Sports Medicine, 1985, p 27.

5   Cai Shijue et al: Tai Ji Quan and the vegetative function of cardiovascular system. 1987's All China Academic Discussion about Wu Shu.

6   Xu Shengwen et al: An observation on respiratory function of aged Tai Ji Quan players. 1964's All China Academic Discussion about Sports Science (abstracts of papers). Division of Sports Physiology and Sports Medicine. Committee of Scientific Work, National Committee of Physical education and Sports, 1964, p 75.

7   Jiang Jianxin: An observation on the effect of Tai Ji Quan on serum HDL-C and other blood lipids. Chin J Sports Med 1984; 3:99.

8   Xu Shengwen, Wang Wenjian: A study of the effect of Tai Ji Quan on endocrinology. Chin J Sports Med 1986; 5:150,

9   Sun Xusheng, et al: E rosette forming test in Tai Ji Quan players. 1986's All China Academic Discussion about Sports Physiology and Sports Biochemistry (abstracts of papers). Chinese Association of Sports Medicine, 1986, p 136.

10 Huang Shijun, et al: Some physiological changes during simplified Tai Ji Quan exercise. 1964's All China Academic Discussion about Sports Science (abstracts of papers). Division of Sports Physiology and Sports Medicine. Committee of Scientific Work, National Committee of Physical Education and Sports, 1964, p 76.

11 Zhuo Dahong: Cardiovascular and respiratory changes during Tai Ji Quan exercise. 1982's All China Academic Discussion about Therapeutic Exercise (abstract of papers). Chinese Association of Sports Medicine, 1982, p 33.

12 Chao Wenyuan: Energy consumption in Tai Ji Quan exercise. 1987's All China Academic Discussion about Wu-Shu.

13   Chen Wenhe, Chao Fusheng: Energy cost of Tai Ji Quan exercise. 1984's All China Aca-
     demic Discussion about Sports Physiology and Sports Medicine (abstracts of papers).
     Chinese Association of Sports Medicine, 1984, p 53.
14   Ju Zhiping, et al: An EEG study on aged Tai Ji Quan players. 1964's All China Academic
     Discussion about Sports Science (abstracts of papers). Division of Sports Physiology and
     Sports Medicine. Committee of Scientific work. National Committee of Physical Educa-
     tion and Sports, 1964, p 76.
15   Hu Huaizhong, et al: An EEG study on famous Tai Ji Quan players. 1987's All China
     Academic discussion about Wu-Shu.

Xu Shengwen, MD, Department of Sports Medicine, Hua-Shan Hospital, Shanghai
Medical University, Shanghai 200040 (China)

Qu Mianyu, Yu Changlong (eds): China's Sports Medicine.
Medicine Sport Sci. Basel, Karger, 1988, vol 28, pp 81–89

Effects of Aerobic Training and Qigong on the Prostacyclin-Thromboxane A₂ Balance of Patients with Coronary Heart Disease

Zhou Shifang, Cao Guohua, Jing Yu, Li Jianan

Department of Sports Medicine and Rehabilitation, Nanjing Medical College, Nanjing, China

Introduction

Prostacyclin (PGI_2) and thromboxane A_2 (TXA_2) are substances which play an important role in the regulation of some physiological processes [1, 2]. The former is so far the strongest vasodilator and platelet disaggregator, and the latter is the strongest vasoconstrictor and platelet aggregator. They are primarily produced by vascular endothelial cells and platelets, respectively.

In recent years, there has been considerable research on the role of PGI_2-TXA_2 imbalance in the etiology, diagnosis and treatment of coronary heart disease (CHD) [3–10]. Some authors had also reported that exercise hat a significant effect on the PGI_2-TXA_2 balance, but most of these experiments aimed at exploring the pathogenesis of ischemic heart disease and almost all of them only observed the acute effects of exercise [11–17]. Knowledge concerning the effects of physical training and static Qigong on the production of PGI_2 or TXA_2 was, however, scanty. Therefore, we studied it and further explored the mechanism of CHD rehabilitation.

Materials and Methods

Subjects

Thirty male CHD patients (mean age 62.6 ± 1.02 years) were equally divided into three groups at random: (1) aerobic training group (mean age 63.8 ± 2.49 years); (2) Qigong group (mean age 62.6 ± 1.63 years) and (3) placebo group (mean age 61.4 ± 0.90 years). Another 10 apparently healthy subjects of similar ages were also studied as the control.

The diagnosis of CHD was based on the history of typical angina pectoris and myocardial infarction combining ECG findings and other laboratory analyses.

Program

The subjects in the aerobic training group and the Qigong group were hospitalized and received aerobic training and static Qigong, while those in the placebo group received placebo only and were dealt with in the out-patient department. The course of treatment was 2 months.

All patients were initially subjected to a graded maximal exercise test in order to determine the maximal heart rate. We used the WHO exercise protocol consisting of continuous 25-watt increments every 2 min starting from 25 W work load. The termination of exercise test was judged by: (1) predicted maximal age-related heart rate (220-age); (2) angina pectoris induced by exercise; (3) the abnormal response of blood pressure and electrocardiogram, and (4) inability to continue exercising because of fatigue or other upsets.

Aerobic exercise was mainly cycling on the ergometer. We used the chronic CHD rehabilitation program which was designed by our department. This program required patients to cycle once a day except Sunday. Every time covered about 40 min consisting of three stages. At stage I, patients first did some relaxed gymnastics and then cycled from 0 W work load with continuous 25-watt increments every 3 min until the patient's heart rate achieved the target heart rate which was 60–80% of the maximum gained by the maximal exercise test. This stage usually lasted about 10 min. At stage II, patients continued cycling at the target heart rate for 20 min. At stage III, the work load was decreased step by step and also required about 10 min.

Static Qigong was carried out collectively in the morning at least once a day and every time covered about 30 min. Usually quiet parks were selected for the Qigong therapy. During the course of practise the patients induce total concentration, and the whole body should be highly relaxed. The breath and heart rate should be very stable, otherwise the patient cannot be considered as being in the Qigong state. In the placebo group, we used the starch, which was taken three times a day and delivered every week. The control healthy subjects did not enter any treatment program.

Measurement of PGI$_2$ and TXA$_2$

All subjects performed the graded submaximal exercise test (terminal heart rate: 195-age). Before and after this test, blood was withdrawn with minimal venous occlusion into the heparinized vacuum tubes containing indomethacin. The plasma was separated immediately by centrifugation (3000 g, 4 C, 15 min), extracted by redistilled acetidin dried by negative pressure and stored at -20 C. Before radioimmunoassay the dried samples were redissolved with BPS, thus PGI production was measured by the concentration of its stable metabolite, immunoreactive 6-keto-prostaglandin Fα (6-K-P) in plasma. The capacity of platelets to produce TXA$_2$ was evaluated by the concentration of its stable metabolite, immunoreactive thromboxane B$_2$(TXB$_2$).

During the course of the experiment, all subjects had not taken any drugs known to interfere with the synthesis of prostaglandins. The determination of plasma 6-K-P and TXB$_2$ level of all CHD patients were carried out again after a period of treatment.

Analysis of variance, followed by t or f tests was used for the statistical analysis.

Results

Before the treatment, the plasma concentration of 6-K-P, TXB$_2$ and the 6-K-P/TXB$_2$ ratio of all CHD patients and healthy subjects are shown in table I. From this table it can be seen that both before and after exercise, the

Table I. The 6-K-P, TXB_2 value and 6-K-P/TXB_2 ratio of CHD patients and normal subjects before therapy

	6-K-P	TXB_2	6-K-P/TXB_2
Control			
Before exercise	199.49 ± 28.05	104.96 ± 13.00	2.02 ± 0.30
After Exercise	174.97 ± 17.46	101.38 ± 20.91	2.06 ± 0.42
CHD			
Before exercise	84.50 ± 7.53**	112.67 ± 8.98	0.86 ± 0.11**
After Exercise	79.80 ± 9.02**	112.70 ± 10.76	0.86 ± 0.09**

** < 0.01 as compared with control group.

Table II. The plasma 6-K-P, TXB_2 level and 6-K-P/TXB_2 ratio of CHD patients before therapy

	Aerobic training	Qigong	Placebo
6-K-P			
Before exercise	70.28 ± 12.05	106.54 ± 15.08	76.70 ± 9.60
After exercise	54.88 ± 8.01	110.55 ± 13.32	73.44 ± 7.21
TXB_2			
Before exercise	106.16 ± 11.47	145.23 ± 12.47	68.17 ± 6.51
After exercise	117.82 ± 23.0	139.62 ± 18.71	80.42 ± 6.51
6-K-P/TXB_2			
Before exercise	0.725 ± 0.138	0.797 ± 0.143	1.145 ± 0.272
After exercise	0.737 ± 0.199	0.907 ± 0.166	0.935 ± 0.086

Table III. The value of plasma 6-K-P, TXB_2 and G-K-P/TXB_2 ratio of CHD patients after a course of treatment

	Aerobic training	Qigong	Placebo
6-K-P			
Before exercise	123.74 ± 17.48**	208.47 ± 36.42**	79.11 ± 14.30
After exercise	79.43 ± 13.47	169.67 ± 31.34**	68.61 ± 15.06
TXB_2			
Before exercise	52.82 ± 7.38*	146.59 ± 25.35*	86.59 ± 13.73
After exercise	77.19 ± 12.27	162.34 ± 43.15*	54.80 ± 5.81
6-K-P/TXB_2			
Before exercise	2.704 ± 0.463**	1.540 ± 0.207*	1.252 ± 0.429
After exercise	1.142 ± 0.152	1.460 ± 0.760*	1.115 ± 0.202

* < 0.05; **p < 0.01, as compared with placebo.

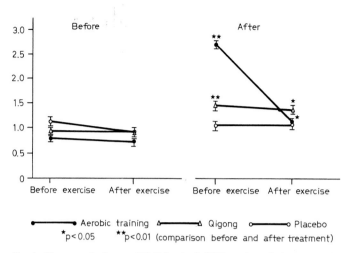

Fig. 1. Changes of plasma 6-K-P level of CHD patients before and after a course of treatment.

plasma 6-K-P level and the 6-K-P/TXB$_2$ ratio of all CHD patients were significantly lower than those of healthy subjects, but the plasma TXB$_2$ levels were the same. Neither CHD patients nor healthy subjects had any changes of plasma 6-K-P, TXB$_2$ and 6-K-P/TXB$_2$ ratio after exercise.

The plasma concentration of 6-K-P, TXB$_2$ and 6-K-P/TXB$_2$ ratio before and after treatment are shown in tables II and III.

Both aerobic training and Qigong for one course significantly increase the plasma 6-K-P level and 6-K-P/TXB$_2$ ratio of CHD patients and aerobic training also decreased the plasma TXB$_2$ level, while in the placebo group there was no alteration of these indices after the course (fig. 1–3). All treatments could not change the response of the patient's PGI$_2$-TXA$_2$ balance to the submaximal exercise.

Discussion

CHD and PGI$_2$-TXA$_2$ Balance

CHD is the result of atherosclerosis of the coronary vessels. The PGI$_2$-TXA$_2$ imbalance, which has been emphasized more and more in recent years, was considered as the key link of development of atherosclerosis. Current

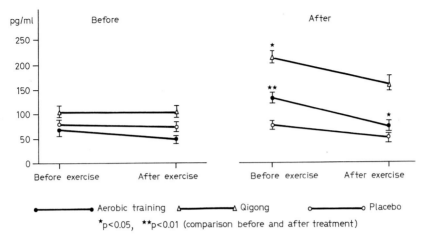

Fig. 2. Changes of plasma TXB$_2$ level of CHD patients before and after a course of treatment.

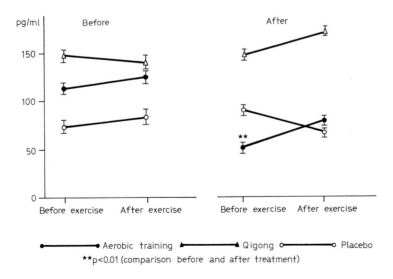

Fig. 3. Change of plasma 6-K-P/TXB$_2$ ratio of CHD patients before and after a course of treatment.

theory holds that atherosclerotic plaque formation damages the histologic and functional integrity of the endothelium. A number of causative factors have been identified in endothelial damage: hemodynamic shearing at bends and bifurcations of the arterial system, low-density lipoproteins (LDL) in the bloodstream, immune complexes and other factors may play a role. It has been postulated that once the intact arterial endothelium is disrupted, plasma components, especially the LDL, are deposited in the denuded area, followed by migration of smooth muscle cells into the subintimal space. At the same time, circulating platelets adhere/aggregate to seal off the injury and release (1) TXA_2 which causes further platelets clumping, thrombosis and vasoconstriction, and (2) a growth factor which stimulates the smooth muscle cells to proliferate in the injured site. Reduced production of PGI_2 at the injured site is overwhelmed by TXA_2 and thus makes the situation worse and worse. There are many reports which suggest that compared to normal subjects, CHD patients have a lower plasma 6-K-P level and 6-K-P/TBX_2 ratio, but a higher plasma TXB_2 concentration [4, 6–9]. Our study agreed with these findings, but the TXB_2 value had not any difference between CHD patients and normal subjects. This may be explained by the different stage of disease. Based on experiments, Risk [13] pointed out that anoxia was an important factor which stimulated the selective release of TXA_2. At the stable stage of chronic CHD, the anoxia is relatively unimportant. Chinese scholars [18] reported the results of circulating TXB_2 level of a group of old CHD patients. Among them 5 cases were acute myocardial infarction, 18 cases were postmyocardial infarction, 23 cases were angina pectoris with frequent attacks, and 15 cases were stable exertional angina pectoris. The value of plasma TXB_2 was compared with 30 normal subjects; only patients who suffered from acute myocardial infarction and frequent attacks of angina pectoris had significantly higher plasma TXB_2 concentrations, while there were no differences in plasma TXB_2 levels among patients suffering from postmyocardial infarction, angina pectoris which was in a stable stage and normal subjects. Most of the CHD patients in our experiment were chronic ones, so similar results were achieved.

PGI_2-TXA_2 Balance and Exercise

Our experiment also suggested that the response of CHD patients' PGI_2-TXA_2 balance to exercise did not agree with other researchers' reports which stated that after exercise plasma PGI_2 did not vary but TXB_2 increased significantly [11, 12]. In our study there were no changes in plasma PGI_2 or

TXA_2 values after submaximal exercise. This, however, was in agreement with the research by Rotmensch et al. [16] in which they found that no changes in the circulating TXB_2 could be detected after exercise either. Although we cannot exclude the possibility of different response to different exercise, one conclusion could be drawn that submaximal ergometer exercise did not induce a PGI_2-TXA_2 imbalance in most chronic CHD patients.

Knowledge about the response of normal subjects' PGI_2-TXA_2 balance to exercise was controversial. Some authors [11] reported that after exercise the plasma 6-K-P level of normal subjects increased, and the TXB_2 remained unchanged. Our study supported Viniikka's [14] findings that before and after exercise the plasma 6-K-P and TXB_2 remained unchanged. The possible explanation for this contradiction lay in the different times of sampling. Viniikka found that plasma 6-K-P was increased at the seventh minute of the exercise test, but not at the end of the exercise or 30 min later. TXB_2 did not change. Our blood samples were all taken at the end of the submaximal exercise test, this may be the reason for the similar results.

Effects of Aerobic Training and Qigong on the PGI_2-TXA_2 Balance of CHD Patients

The plasma 6-K-P level and 6-K-P/TXB_2 ratio were significantly increased, but TXB_2 decreased after a course of treatment. This suggests that aerobic training of about 2 months has a beneficial influence on the PGI_2-TXA_2 balance. We suppose this influence may be indirect. A lot of experiments confirmed that exercise can decrease heart rate, blood pressure and increase the cardiac output, thus improving the oxygen supply to the tissues [19–22] and inhibiting the selective release of TXA_2 due to anoxia. In addition, exercise elevated the plasma HDL level, reduced LDL [23–25], while HDL can enhance the synthesis of PGI_2 and LDL can interfere with it. HDL inhibits the platelet aggregation [26, 27], which also slows down the release of TXA_2.

Qigong therapy is one of the valuable heritages of Chinese traditional medicine. The blood pressure of a Qigong practician had a regular varied pattern during practising [28]. In the Qigong state, the ECG of the practician had a special change-synchronization of the α-wave [29]. Static Qigong of 2 months can significantly increase the plasma 6-K-P level and 6-K-P/TXB_2 ratio, but cannot change the TXB_2. This suggests that Qigong can influence the synthesis of PGI_2 within the endothelium by its active protective function.

Conclusion

We conclude that prescribed aerobic exercise, which is based on the result of a graded maximal exercise test, generally does not interfere with the balance of PGI_2-TXA_2 in vivo and both aerobic training and Qigong have the beneficial effects on the PGI_2-TXA_2 system, so they can be effectively used in the rehabilitation of CHD patients.

References

1   Hamberg M, et al: Thromboxane. A new group of biologically active compounds derived from prostaglandin endoperoxide. Proc Natl Acad Sci USA 1975; 72:2994.

2   Moncada S, et al: An enzyme isolated from arteries transformed prostaglandin endoperoxides to an unstable substance that inhibited platelet aggregation. Nature 1976; 263:663.

3   Tada M, et al: Elevation of thromboxane B_2 levels in patients with classic and variant angina pectoris. Circulation 1981; 64:1107.

4   Numano F, et al: Coronary spasm, prostaglandin and HLA factors. Jpn Circ J 1985; 49:119.

5   Friedrich T, et al: Follow-up of prostaglandin plasma levels after acute myocardial infarction. Am Heart J 1985; 109:218.

6   Robertson RM, et al: Thromboxane A_2 in vasotonic angina pectoris. Evidence from direct measurement and inhibitor trails. New Engl J Med 1981: 304:998.

7   Jouve R, et al: Thromboxane B_2 6-keto-PGF, α, PGE_2, $PGF_2\alpha$, PGA, plasma levels in arteriosclerosis obliterans: Relationship to clinical manifestations, risk factors and arterial pathanatomy. Am Heart J 1984: 107:45.

8   Fitzgerald GA, et al: Increased prostacyclin biosynthesis in patients with severe atherosclerosis and platelet activation. New Engl J Med 1984; 310:1068.

9   Yamazaki H, et al: Thromboxane A_2 synthetizing activity of platelets in acute myocardial infarction. Blood & Vessels 1984; 15:149.

10   Ganz P, et al: Effects of prostacyclin on coronary hemodynamics at rest and in response to cold pressor testing in patients with angina pectoris. Am J Cardiol 1984: 53:1500.

11   Mehta J, et al: The significance of platelet-vessel wall prostaglandin equilibrium during exercise-induced stress. Am Heart J 1983; 105:895.

12   Yazima M, et al: Plasma thromboxane B_2, 6-keto-PGI_2 and cyclic nucleotides levels as related to treadmill exercise test in patients with ischemic heart disease. Jap Circ J 1985; 49:38.

13   Risk C, et al: Thromboxane and prostacyclin(epoprostenol) during exercise in diffuse pulmonary fibrosis. Lancet 1982; 11:1183.

14   Viniikka L.: Lipid peroxides, prostacyclin and thromboxane A_2 in runners during acute exercise. Med Sci Sports Exerc 1984; 18:275.

15   Siess W, et al: Plasma catecholamines, platelet aggregation and associated thromboxane formation after physical exercise, smoking or norepinephrine infusion. Circulation 1982; 66:48.

16   Rotmensch HH, et al: Plasma platelet products and exercise-induced myocardial ischemia. J Lab Clin Med 1983; 102:63.
17   Yamamoto, et al : Effects of treadmill exercise test on prostacyclin in patients with exertional angina pectoris. Resp Circul (Jap) 1984; 32:105.
18   Shen Wenjing, et al: The clinical value of detection of TXB_2 in patients with coronary heart disease. Personal communication 1986.
19   Cantwell JD: Exercise and coronary heart disease. Role in primary prevention. Heart Lung 1984; 13:6.
20   Froelicher V, et al: Cardiac rehabilitation; Evidence for improvement in myocardial perfusion and function. Arch Phys Med Rehabil 1980; 61:517.
21   Ehsani AA, et al: Cardiac effects of prolonged and intense exercise training in patients with coronary artery disease. Am J Cardio 1982; 50:246.
22   Longhurst JC, et al: Chronic training with static and dynamic exercise: Cardiovascular adaptation and response to exercise. Circ Res 1981; 48:1171.
23   Health GW, et al: Exercise training improves lipoprotein lipid profiles in patients with coronary artery disease. Am Heart J 1983; 105:839.
24   Cowan GO: Influence of exercise on high-density lipoproteins. Am J Cardiol 1983; 52:138.
25   Thompson PD, et al: Exercise, diet or physical characteristics as determinants of HDL levels in endurance athletes. Atherosclerosis 1983; 46:333.
26   Aviram M, et al: Platelet interaction with high and low density lipoproteins. Atherosclerosis 1983; 46:259.
27   Khalfen, et al: Effects of different classes of lipoprotein on platelet aggregation (abstract). Cardiologia (Russ) 1984, 2:32
28   Wang Galing, et al: Experimental observation of the changes of blood pressure during Qigong state. Nature (Chin) 1980; 3:743.
29   Mei-Lei, et al: The research of electric wave in Qigong state. Nature (Chin) 1981; 4:662.

Zhou Shifang, MD, Department of Sports Medicine and Rehabilitation, Nanjing Medical College, Nanjing (China)

Qu Mianyu, Yu Changlong (eds): China's Sports Medicine.
Medicine Sport Sci. Basel, Karger, 1988, vol 28, pp 90–93

Effect of Acupuncture on Ultrastructural Alteration in Skeletal Muscle after Strenuous Exercise[1]

Lu Dinghou[a], Duan Changping[a], Zhang Jianguo[a], Fan Jingyu[b],
Tang Xiaojing[c]

[a] Section of Exercise Physiology and Institute of Physical Education; [b] Section of
Biophysics, Beijing Medical University; [c] Plant Biochemistry Lab, Beijing Agriculture
University, Beijing, China

Sports injuries of the skeletal muscles incurred during training are common in athletes. They seriously affect the athletes' ability to work and to carry out their daily training. As these injuries are likely to be associated closely with the accumulation of ultrastructural changes within the muscles resulting from strenuous exercise, it would be of great significance both theoretically and practically to research into the factors which govern the ultrastructural and functional changes after a heavy work load and to find an effective treatment which would contribute to quicken the recovery process.

*Ultrastructural and Functional Changes of the Skeletal Muscle after
Strenuous Exercise*

Unaccustomed or strenuous exercise often leads to delayed-onset muscle soreness. Reduction in contractility and flexibility and increase in muscle stiffness very much resemble the symptoms of some sports injures of the skeletal muscle and must be related to the ultrastructural changes within the muscle fiber. So, close observation of the ultrastructural changes of skeletal

[1] Projects supported by the Science Fund of the Chinese Academy of Sciences.

muscle after strenuous exercise might be an important way of approaching the investigation of the mechanisms of some sports injuries of the skeletal muscle.

In recent years, Chinese researchers already observed structural changes of the cell membrane, nucleus, mitochondria, lysosome, myofibril and myofibrillar filament in skeletal muscles after strenuous exercise, but we mainly focused our attention on the ultrastructural changes related to the contraction and relaxation of the skeletal muscle.

Among the findings from our observations are: changed arrangement of the myofibril; sarcomeres are shortened or of irregular lengths; Z lines streamed or broadened and those in the sarcomeres partially or totally disappeared; structure of myofibrillar filament notably changed or totally disappeared.

By immunoelectron-microscopic observation of the myosin thick filament in skeletal muscles after a heavy work load, we found that immune reactions still exist as long as the structure of the thick filaments remains; however, an immune reaction no longer exists as the thick filament structure disappears [5].

Ultrastructural changes and focal disappearance of structures in myofibrils invariably affect the contractility and flexibility of the muscles.

Acupuncture Facilitates the Recovery Process of Ultrastructural Changes in Skeletal Muscles after Strenuous Exercise

Qualitative analysis, made by Duan Changping [2] by way of electron-microscopic observations of biopsies from vastus lateralis muscles of subject 24 h after heavy squatting-jumping exercise shows that prominent focal structural changes took place in the myofibril of the vastus lateralis muscles of subjects without acupuncture treatment, while no such prominent changes or approximate to normal conditions were registered in biopsies from the other legs of the same subjects when treated with acupuncture. The results of the observations indicate that acupuncture serves either to inhibit the process of changes in protein of the myofibril, or to promote the process of recovery.

Quantitative analysis made by Zhang Jianguo [3] by means of electron-microsocopic observations of biopsies from the vastus lateralis muscles of 4 subjects 24 h after heavy squatting exercise shows that 68.15% of the Z lines under observation were streamed or disappeared in the myofibril of the leg without acupuncture treatment, while only 38.9% were registered in the straightly acupunctured leg and 31.23% were registered in the obliquely acupunctured leg. The difference of rates of changes in the Z lines between those with and without acupuncture treatment is prominent statistically (< 0.01). The difference of rates of changes in the Z lines between those acupunctured straightly or obliquely is also prominent statistically (< 0.01). Furthermore, both ways of acupuncture serve to reduce the amount of myofibrillar filament involved in the changes after heavy work load considerably; the volume density of the changed myofibrillar tissues was 9.44% in those without acupuncture and 0.27% in those straightly acupunctured, but no myofibrillar changes were observed in those acupunctured obliquely.

These findings not only confirmed that acupuncture greatly helps the recovery process of protein in myofibrils in skeletal muscles after heavy work load, but also provide preliminary scientific evidence in support of the ancient prescription that ailments of the muscle should be treated with acupuncture obliquely, as is stated in the classic Chinese medical book *Lingshujing*.

Acupuncture (Oblique) Is Effective in the Treatment of
Sports Injuries in Skeletal Muscles

For more than the last 10 years, we have applied oblique acupuncture for the treatment of strains or tears muscle cramps such as strain of the lower back muscles, severe cramp of the soleus, injury of the piriform muscle, and patients suffering from chronic muscle problems resulting from overuse of their muscles, and have achieved good results. For example, among the 140 cases in 1981 to which acupuncture treatment was applied, 118 were cured (symptoms disappeared, function restored), which comprises 84.28% of the total cases, and 20 cases, or 14.29% of the total, registered marked recovery. By the end of 1985, a number of Chinese elite short-track speedskaters (male and female) suffered from muscle stiffness and soreness, which greatly affected their coordination of movements, preventing them from further training. They recovered, however, soon after oblique acupuncture treatment. During 1985–1986, 4 javelin throwers suspended their training because of pain in the elbow, which, too, was soon relieved after oblique acupuncture treatment was administered in collaboration with the coach, and their training was resumed.

Summary

Skeletal muscle injuries are common in athletes, which is likely to be closely associated with accumulation of ultrastructural alterations within the skeletal muscles resulting from strenuous exercise. We focused our main attention in this area. By ways of qualitative and quantitative electron-microscopic observations of biopsies from vastus lateralis muscle after strenuous exercise, we found that acupuncture, especially the oblique method, serves either to inhibit the process of changes in the protein content of the myofibrils or to promote the process of their recovery. For more than the last 10 years, we have applied oblique acupuncture for the treatment of a series of sports injuries of the skeletal muscle and achieved good results.

References

1   Lu Ding Hou: Effect of acupuncture on relieving muscle spasm. Symposium of 30th Anniversary of Beijing Institute of Physical Education; 1st part, pp 120–122 (1983).

2   Duan Changping: Effect of acupuncture and static stretch on the ultrastructural alterations of skeletal muscle during delayed onset muscle soreness. J Beijing Inst Phys Educ 1984; 4:8–19.

3   Zhang Jianguo: Effect of acupuncture (straight and oblique) on the ultrastructural alterations post strenuous oblique-squat exercise China Sports Sci. Soci 1988; 1:61–64.

4   Lin Yuwen: Effect of acupuncture on relaxing the skeletal muscle of swimmer. J Beijing Inst Phys Educ 1982; 4:73–76.

5   Lu Dinghou; Fan Jingyu; Tang Xiaojing: An immunoelectron-microscopic observation of the structural alteration of myosin filament after strenuous exercise (unpublished data).

Lu Dinghou, MD, Beijing Institute of Physical Education,
Beijing 100084 (China)

Qu Mianyu, Yu Changlong (eds): China's Sports Medicine.
Medicine Sport Sci. Basel, Karger, 1988, vol 28, pp 94–113

Some Sports Nutrition Researches in China

Ji Di Chen

Research Division of Sports Nutrition and Biochemistry, Institute of Sports Medicine,
Beijing Medical University, Beijing, China

Physical exercise is an important aid to keep people fit, but it also enhances the metabolic process of the body; therefore, problems of sports nutrition deserve consideration.

Research on the Nutrition Metabolism and Requirement of Athletes

Most sport events require high energy expenditure because of the great intensity and oxygen debt [1–3]. The energy metabolism rate of exercise may be several and even a hundred times more than that of a sedentary state (table I). The data of an hour's exercise energy expenditure in training was compared with that of the classified degree of physical labor in China [4], it is clearly seen that the energy expenditure of the majority of sport events corresponds to that of the heavy and heaviest labor, and sometimes even more (table II). Energy requirements of athletes are closely related to physical load including the intensity, density, and the duration of exercise. Investigation of the energy expenditure of the ten sport events showed that the requirement of the majority sports were mostly in the range of 3,500–4,400 kcal/day, the data correspond to the RDA of heavy or the heaviest laboring people in China as given by the Health Institute of the Chinese Academy of Medical Sciences (tables III, IV). Recently, research on the correlation of energy expenditure and heart rates has been conducted on Chinese dancers including ballet, orient dance, centre dance, and song and drama dance [5]. The intensity of protein metabolism of athletes is much higher than sedentary people. The 24 h urinary creatinine excretions were 1.5–2.0 times that of normal persons [6]. When the exercise load was augmented, the energy intake was increased correspondingly, and as the protein

Table I. Energy expenditure and relative metabolic rate (RMR) of different sport events

Sport events	Energy expenditure rate kcal/kg/min	RMR
Yang's Taijiquan (Chinese boxing)	0.1002 ± 0.0022	4.3
Wu's Taijiquan (Chinese boxing)	0.0814 ± 0.0079	3.3
Shao-lingquan (Chinese boxing)	0.1914 ± 0.0171	9.3
Acrobatic gymnastics	2.0999 ± 0.0228	112.4
Weight-lifting snatch 90 kg	2.1399 ± 0.2708	133.0
Motor cycling handicapped	0.1382 ± 0.0130	6.4

Energy expenditure rate of rest, 0.0191 ± 0.0014 kcal/kg/min.

$$RMR = \frac{\text{Energy expenditure of exercise} - \text{energy expenditure of rest}}{\text{Basal metabolic rate}}$$

Table II. Energy expenditures during the training period of athletes compared with general people

Sport events	Mean energy expenditure		
	kcal/h	kcal/kg/h	kcal/m² body surface/h
Swimming, throwing	> 600	> 7.0	> 300
Basketball, volleyball, weight-lifting, motorcycling, radiodirector finding	> 300	> 5.0	> 200
Weight-lifting (flyweight), model of navigation, table tennis, radio	150–300	> 3.0	> 100

The mean energy expenditure of Chinese people are as follows:

Light	physical labor	120 kcal/h
Moderate	physical labor	170 kcal/h
Heavy	physical labor	270 kcal/h
The most heavy	physical labor	370 kcal/h

intake was kept the same, the urinary nitrogen output increased significantly from 10.0 ± 0.34 to 12.7 ± 0.34 g/day, it was about 20% greater (fig. 1). Based on the research of the estimated nitrogen balance experiments, the protein requirement of adult athletes averaged 1.8–2.4 g/kg body weight, and it was 3.0 g/kg for children and 2.0 g/kg for juvenile athletes. The requirement was suggested to increase to 3.3 g/kg for children in amateur training with low intakes of animal foods and 2.5 g/kg for juveniles in intensive training, respectively. As the diet control measures were adopted to reduce the body weight of athletes, the energy from protein food source should be increased to 17–19% of the total (table V).

The differences between water and mineral metabolism of athletes training under normal temperature and that of average sedentary people are not significant, but the condition would change during exercise in a hot environment with sweat losses increasing markedly. In long-distance running in a temperature of 24–31.5 °C, the volume of sweat output was 1,617–3,495 ml, which was 2.9–6.0% of the body weight and 699–846 ml/h/m² of body surface area. The excretion of sweat NaCl and potassium amount were high. The total output of NaCl reached the amount of 18–22 g/day. NaCl and potassium balance were both in a negative state (table VI; fig. 2). The high-

Table III. Energy expenditure and requirement of different sport events

Sport events	Sex	Mean energy Expenditure kcal/day	Mean energy requirement kcal/day	Mean energy requirement kcal/kg
Swimming	M	3,831	4,406	63
	F	2,976	3,422	58
Basketball	M	3,906	4,492	53
	F	3,200	3,680	63
Volleyball	M	3,688	4,141	53
	F	3,510	4,037	62
Table tennis	M	3,192	3,671	56
	F	2,648	3,045	53
Throwing	M	4,572	5,258	54
	F	3,672	4,223	49
Weight-lifting	M			
Heavy weight		4,155	4,778	44
Feather weight		2,804	3,225	52
Flyweight		2,266	2,602	45
Motorcycling	M	3,677	4,229	58
	F	3,101	3,556	58

Table IV. RDA of energy in China

Degree of physical labor	Energy allowance, kcal/day male	Energy allowance, kcal/day female
Extremely light	2,400	2,200
Light	2,600	2,400
Moderate	3,000	2,800
Heavy	3,600	3,400
Heaviest	4,200	–

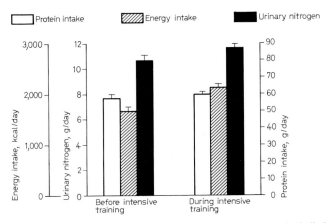

Fig. 1. The change of urinary nitrogen excretion of amateur basketball players before and during intensive training.

Table V. Protein requirement of athletes under different conditions

Sport events	Age	Sex	Conditions	Protein g/day	Requirement g/kg
Weight-lifting	adult	male	moderate erxercise	148 ± 2.8	2.36 ± 0.21
Gymnastics	adult	male	before competition	118 ± 4.2	1.92 ± 0.07
Gymnastics	children	male	growth and development period (amateur training)	79 ± 2.1	3.09 ± 0.08
Basketball	juvenile	female	growth and development period (amateur training)	92 ± 3.3	2.00 ± 0.07
Gymnastics	children	male	training with a lowered nutrition diet	86 ± 3.9	3.35 ± 0.15
Basketball	juvenile	female	increased physical training load	116 ± 3.9	2.52 ± 0.08
Gymnastics	adult	female	weight reduction period before competition	97 ± 8.2	1.80 ± 0.15

Table VI. Volume and mineral content of athletes sweat running in a hot environment

Distance of running m	Num- ber	Temp °C	RH %	Volume of sweat		Mineral content of sweat, g	
				ml	% of body weight	NaCl	K
30,000	4	31.5	74	2,565 ± 497	4.53 ± 0.89	12.83 ± 2.49	2.95 ± 0.40
30,000	5	26.0	73	2,230 ± 470	3.95 ± 0.97	11.15 ± 2.35	3.44 ± 0.98
42,195	5	24.0	84	2,786 ± 501	4.92 ± 0.82	13.88 ± 2.50	–

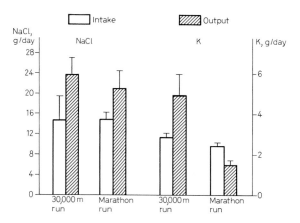

Fig. 2. Status of the NaCl and K balance of athletes training in hot environments.

Table VII. Tentative RDA of daily minerals for athletes

Condition	K	NaCl	Ca	Mg	Fe
	g/day	g/day	g/day	mg/day	mg/day
Training	3	15	0.8	300–500	15
Competition	4–6	20	1–1.5	500–800	20–25

est value of potassium in sweat was 5.2 g/day. The research results indicated that the mineral requirements of athletes training in hot environments cannot be satisfied by normal intake of minerals. Requirement of NaCl and potassium of athletes training in normal temperatures are 15 and 3 g/day, respectively. Supplementation for athletes training in hot environments should be considered. The amount of supplement may be estimated according to the physical load and sweat losses [7]. Requirement of NaCl and potassium are suggested to be 20 and 4–6 g/day, respectively, for athletes training in hot environments. The requirement of iron has been increased to 20–25 mg/day considering the incidence of iron deficiency anemia was rather high, and iron loss of sweat may be one of the causes of iron deficiency. On the basis of nutrition surveys and blood calcium data, a suggested allowance of dietary Ca 1 g/day is recommended (table VII).

Research on the vitamin C metabolism of organism in exercise illustrated that vitamin C metabolism is intensified and requirement is increased in exercise. The experimental results showed that blood vitamin C of athletes

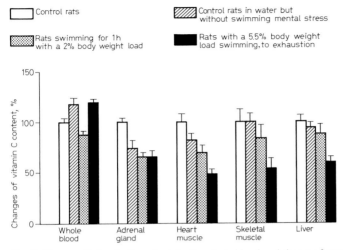

Fig. 3. Change of vitamin C contents in the whole blood and tissues of rats after mental and exercise load in comparison with the control.

Table VIII. Changes in the whole blood vitamin C of subjects after different physical loads

Physical load	Number of cases	Vitamin C, mg%		
		before exercise	after exercise	differ- ence*
Go up and down stairs 30 times/min	11	0.68 ± 0.06	0.83 ± 0.08	+0.15
Go up and down stairs 100 times/5 min	15	0.70 ± 0.04	0.84 ± 0.04	+0.14
Go up and down stairs 200 times/10 min	14	0.67 ± 0.04	0.78 ± 0.09	+0.11
15 sec run at maximum speed	33	0.53 ± 0.03	0.61 ± 0.03	+0.08
3 min run in place (160 steps/min)	17	0.57 ± 0.04	0.73 ± 0.04	+0.16
1,500 m run (moderate speed)	28	0.48 ± 0.04	0.60 ± 0.04	+0.12

*$p < 0.05$.

all increased after different exercises of short duration (table VIII). Animal experiments showed that the increase in blood vitamin C after exercise may be attributed to the mobilization of the vitamin C in the tissues and organs of the body (fig. 3). The vitamin C content of the tissues recovered at 48 h after exercise. It is clear that physical exercise does enhance vitamin C metabolism and consume certain amounts of vitamin C in the tissues and organs [8]. Based on the surveys and estimations of blood and urinary

Table IX. Tentative suggested "RDA" of daily vitamins for athletes (mg/day)

Condition	V_A	Carotene	VB_1	VB_2	V_{pp}	Vc
Training	2	3	3–5	2	20–25	100–150
Competition	2–3	2–3	5–10	2.5	25–30	150–200

Table X. Serum Zn and Cu levels of elite athletes and medical students

Group	Zn		Cu	
	n_o	levels, $\mu g \cdot dl^{-1}$	n_o	levels, $\mu g \cdot dl^{-1}$
Athletes	212	96 ± 19.2*	165	112 ± 18.8*
Medical students	48	108 ± 15.5	52	103 ± 16.2

*p < 0.01. Data of athletes Vs medical students

Table XI. Evaluation of the serum Zn levels of elite athletes

Season	Sex	Number investigated	Number with deficiency	% of deficiency
Spring	male	83	3	3.6
	female	29	0	0
Winter	male	84	8	9.5
	female	128	16	12.5

vitamins for athletes over the years [9], tentative daily requirement of vitamins of athletes has been suggested in table IX. It shows that the majority of the vitamin amounts of athletes were about twofold that of heavy laborers in China [10].

Concern has been drawn to the trace element nutrition for athletes in recent years. Although the average daily intakes of Zn and Cu levels of elite athletes were two times or even more than the RDA of sedentary healthy persons, the incidence of low serum Zn and Cu was still high (tables X, XI) which suggested that the requirement of trace elements might be higher than that of sedentary persons, and further research is needed.

The All China Sports Federation pays close attention to the health and nutritional status of athletes, high level nutrition has been provided for

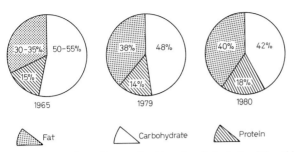

Fig. 4. Energy from diet protein, fat, and carbohydrate of the athletes.

Table XII. Distribution of the blood vitamin C content in 67 athletes

Sport events	Number examined	Blood vitamin C, mg%			
		< 0.4	0.4–0.6	0.6–0.8	> 0.8
Basketball	44	4	6	14	20
Weight-lifting	16	–	–	4	12
Gymnastics	7	–	–	3	4
Total	67	4	6	21	36
% of the total number		6	9	31	54

Table XIII. Distribution of the 4-hour urinary vitamin B_2 output of 175 athletes after taking a dosage of 5 mg

Output of urinary vitamin B_2 in 4 h, µg	Number of cases	% of the total number
< 400	18	10.3
400–800	44	25.1
> 800	113	64.6

athletes in training. Serious nutritional deficiency diseases of athletes cannot be found in China nowadays. Protein intake of athletes has been reaching 1.5–3.0 g/kg. Protein from animal source was greater than 50% of the total for athletes in training, but owing to the lack of reasonable arrangements, nutritional problems still exist. Food fat has been high in athletes' diet, energy from fat source has been increasing to 38–40% of the total (fig. 4),

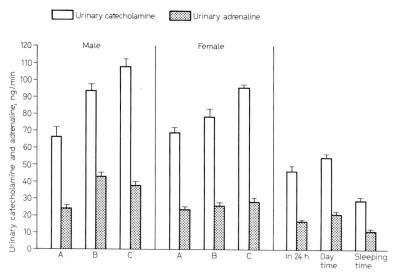

Fig. 5. The excretion of urinary catecholamine of athletes in different functional status compared with the data in the sedentary condition. A = Normal; B = abnormal in one test; C = abnormal in two tests.

and thus carbohydrate was decreased, and some of the athletes were diagnosed to be in hyperlipemia. There have also been existing problems of the inadequacy of vitamins (tables XII, XIII), but these problems are constantly being improved.

Research on the Functional Evaluation of Athletes

On the purpose of diagnosing the early stage of overtraining and dysfunction of athletes, researches on the functional evaluation in the biochemistry of athletes have been developed in China. Synthetic indices including urinary catecholamine [11], blood lactic acid, serum protein [12], and immunoglobin [13] together with heart rate, blood pressure, ECG, etc., were studied. It has been found that the urinary catecholamine output of athletes in rest conditions were comparatively stable, its mean value in sleeping time was 29 ± 2.1 ng/min, and it was 46.8 ± 2.6 ng/min in 24 h. The urinary catecholamine excretion increased promptly after exercise load. There was a tendency towards greater urinary catecholamine excretions in those with

Table XIV. Serum protein components of athletes in different conditions (%) (n = 16)

Functional condition	Pre-exercise				
	albumin	globulin			
		α1	α2	β	γ
Good	70.3 ± 3.6	2.2 ± 0.7	4.6 ± 1.6*	9.3 ± 1.4	13.6 ± 2.5**
Bad	72.5 ± 4.1	2.0 ± 1.2	3.8 ± 1.5*	10.4 ± 2.0	11.3 ± 2.1**
Functional condition	Post-exercise				
	albumin	globulin			
		α1	α2	β	γ
Good	69.0 ± 2.9	2.34 ± 1.0	5.4 ± 1.4**	9.1 ± 1.1	13.5 ± 2.4**
Bad	71.0 ± 3.5	2.62 ± 1.3	4.1 ± 1.2**	10.3 ± 1.8	11.8 ± 2.4**

*Data compared between good and bad conditions showed significance: * < 0.05; ** < 0.01.

higher blood lactic acid, blood pressure, heart rate and myocardial oxygen consumption (fig. 5). Research results showed that most of the changes in the cardiovascular system are closely related to urinary catecholamine in submaximal exercise load.

Acid metabolites accumulate in strenuous exercise. Blood lactic acid increased distinctly after exercise. It was found that athletes having higher blood lactic acid levels after a submaximal exercise were also proved to be in bad functional states. Changes in blood lactic acid ran slightly parallel with urinary catecholamine, their correlation coefficient was + 0.21.

Research results indicated that the serum protein, immunoglobin, blood vitamin C contents and phagocytic activity of the WBC varied under different conditions of athletes. Serum globulin α_2 and γ levels decreased as the conditions of athletes were getting worse and they increased as the conditions got better (table XIV); the serum immunoglobin IgG and IgA levels decreased in overtrained athletes as well (table XV). Vitamin C levels of overtrained athletes were low, the phagocytic activity of their WBC decreased significantly too [14]. Different contents of blood vitamin C of athletes had distinct responses on the phagocytic activity of WBC. The phagocytic activity of WBC was high when vitamin C nutrition was good, otherwise, as vitamin C nutrition status was bad, the phagocytic activity was low (table XVI, fig. 6).

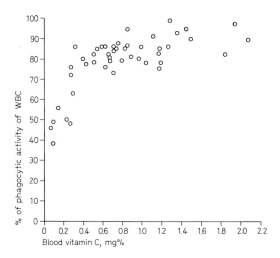

Fig. 6. The relationship between the phagocytic activity of WBC and vitamin C contents of athletes.

Table XV. Serum immunoglobin contents of athletes in normal and overtrained condition

Subject	n	IgG mg/ml	IgA mg/ml	IgM mg/ml
Athletes (normal)	82	12.43 ± 3.25	1.64 ± 0.74*	1.36 ± 0.49
Athletes (overtrained)	15	9.83 ± 2.38*	1.52 ± 0.56*	0.96 ± 0.17
Normal persons	50	12.00 ± 2.62	2.00 ± 0.50	1.10 ± 0.30

*Data compared with normal persons showed significance: * < 0.05.

Table XVI. Phagocytic activity of white blood cells of athletes in different vitamin C status

Athletic condition	Group	Number of cases	Blood vitamin C mg%	% of phagocytic activity
Normal	I	16	1.39 ± 0.09	87 ± 1.74
	II	18	0.76 ± 0.02	84 ± 1.48
	III	8	0.41 ± 0.04	77 + 2.46
Overtrained		6	0.15 ± 0.03	48 ± 3.07

Difference compared group I with II showed no significance: p > 5 %.
Difference compared group I with III showed significance: p < 5 %.
Difference compared group II with III showed significance: p < 5 %.

Research on Nutrition and Its Relation to Sports Anemia

Anemia is a common disease in athletes [15]. Anemia not only debilitates the physical work capacity and training effect of athletes, it also affects the development and growth of children and adolescents; moreover, it is also an inducing factor of overtraining and infectious diseases in athletes. The relation between anemia and physical exercise and nutrition of athletes has brought extensive attention in China. Research results on sports anemia in the past were controversial. Some of the authors attributed the drop in HB and HCT of athletes at the early stage of training to the dilution effect of expanded plasma volume rather than an anemic effect per se, that is the destruction of RBCs. Anyhow, it should be noted that the plasma volume was not actually measured.

The etiology of sports anemia is still not entirely clear. We found that some of the anemic cases in athletes were attributed to some primary diseases, and some of them were induced by intensive exercise and diagnosed to be iron deficiency anemia. Among the cases investigated, regardless of age, iron deficiency anemia appeared to be the major type.

The anemia incidence of adult athletes was found to be 4.9% and it was 15.9% in amateur children and juvenile athletes. It showed that there was a trend towards higher anemia incidences in those of low age groups. Examination of blood revealed that about half of the cases were hypochromic and microcytic iron deficiency anemia, the others were normochromic [15] (tables XVII, XVIII). Since HB levels of athletes are related to multiple factors including physical exercise load and conditioning, so it needs concrete analysis (table XIX).

Studies have recently been conducted on the effects of different exercise load on the deformability and viscosity of RBC. It was found that anaerobic exercise load affects the deformability and viscosity of RBC (table XX), (fig 7, 8).

Table XVII. Anemia incidence in athletes

Groups	Age	Total cases	Number of anemia	Incidence of anemia %
Athletes of College	adult	141	7	4.97
Athletes of training team	adult	169	8	4.91
Amateur athletes	children juvenile	390	62	15.90

Table XVIII. Anemia incidence of different age groups of athletes

Age group	Number of total cases	Number with anemia	Incidence of anemia %
8–10	30	13	43.3
11–12	86	26	30.2
13–14	100	19	19.3
15–16	133	4	3.0

There was no anemia in the age groups over 16 years.
Difference of the anemia incidence among the age groups showed significance, $p < 0.01$.
Difference of the anemia incidence between 8–10 and 11–12 years age groups showed no significance, $p > 0.05$.
Difference of the anemia incidence between 11–12 and 13–14 years age group showed no significance, $p > 0.05$.

Table XIX. Effect of intensive exercise training on the hemoglobin content of athletes

Sport items	n	Pretraining	After 1 month of training	After 2 month of training	t test of the difference between pre- and posttraining
Running	12	13.4 ± 1.43	12.1 ± 0.94	11.5 ± 1.21	$p < 0.05$
Track and field	19	14.6 ± 1.28	13.4 ± 1.18	13.3 ± 1.00	$p < 0.05$
Swimming	9	14.3 ± 1.06	12.9 ± 1.51	–	$p < 0.05$
Basketball	5	11.2 ± 0.94	12.0 ± 1.54	–	$p > 0.05$

Table XX. RBC filter rate and osmotic fragility test bevore and after 100 m sprint (n = 6)

RBC	Filter rate %	osm fragility (NaCl%)
Before	20.7 ± 5.7	0.426 + 0.026
After	10.5 ± 2.3*	0.583 ± 0.046*

*$p < 0.01$.

Research on Special Nutrition Problems of Athletes

Wrestlers, lifters, judo players, and light-weight crew (those who compete at established weight classes) are the special athletic population who often follow weight reduction procedures to 'make weight' for competition; and most athletes lose their weight primarily by partial starvation, fluid restriction, sweating induced by thermal and/or exercise, and diuresis. Stu-

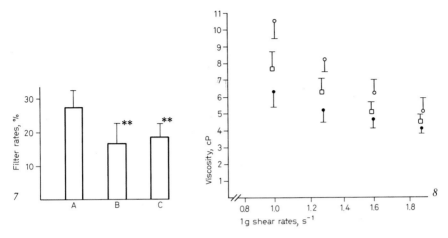

Fig. 7. RBC filter rates of athletes: A = data at rest; B = data immediately after the Wingate test; C = data at 1 h after the Wingate test. Differences between the data at rest and that after the Wingate test were significant: **p < 0.01.

Fig. 8. RBC suspension viscosity of 6 college students decreased in all 4 shear rates immediately after the Wingate test (□), differences of the data and that of the rest (o) was significant, p < 0.05. RBC suspension viscocity decreased continuously at 1 h after exercise (●), differences between the data and that of the data immediately after the Wingate test were significant, p < 0.05.

dies have shown that 3–10% or even more of the pre-competition weight was lost before official certification [16].

Gymnasts, ballet dancers, divers, and distance runners are among the leanest athletes, but they still often attempt to lose or control weight. These athletes primarily adopt a long-term low-calorie diet to control weight, but they also use dehydration, and practices as diuresis, laxatives, or even appetite depressant measures to reach the unrealistic weight goal for competition [17]. Reasons were as follows: lower weight possesses some biomechanical advantages in sports with body moving or lifting; to achieve a maximum ratio of muscle strength to body weight; additional weight requires extra strength and energy in sports, and sometimes it may be a factor in inhibiting success, especially in intensive and competitive performance; and gymnasts and dancers always want to keep their body slim and are overly aware of their body shape. Unfortunately, the most commonly used practices of either rapid weight reduction or long-term weight control both cause health problems and impairment of physical capacity.

(1) Health problems induced by rapid weight loss are as follows:
(a) Body water loss – dehydration (table XXI).
(b) Increased load on cardiovascular system. Body fluid loss leads to reduced cardiac output, smaller stroke volume, a lower oxygen uptake and a reduction in cardiac functioning during submaximal work loads associated with higher heart rates (table XXII).

Table XXI. Effects of weight reduction (WR) on the hemoglobin and blood glucose concentration of lifters

Number of cases	Hemoglobin, g%		Blood glucose, mg%	
	pre.WR	post-WR	pre-WR	post-WR
12	14.7 ± 1.16	16.1 ± 1.49	101 ± 13.5	104 ± 20.5
t test	$p < 0.05$		$p > 0.05$	

Table XXII. Effects of weight reduction on the BP, P and pulse pressure of lifters

Athlete group	Number of cases	BP, mm/Hg		
		pre-WR	WR	post-WR
Control (no weight reduction)	5		118 + 8.2/ 79 ± 7.6	
Experimental (weight reduction)	8	112 ± 4.9/ 72 ± 10.2		102 ± 13[1,3]/ 70 + 10[2]

Difference between pre and post weight reduction showed significance, [1]$p < 0.05$.
Difference between lifters with or without weight reduction showed significance, [2]$p < 0.05$, and obvious significance [3]$p < 0.01$.

Table XXIII. Effects of weight reduction on the urine volume of lifters

Time	Case. No.	Volume of 24-hours urine, ml	
		pre-WR	post-WR
1980.4	8	1.006 ± 52	469 ± 103**
1980.10	7	1.087 ± 272	503 ± 173**
1981.5	4	771 ± 195	559 ± 262*

Differences in the 24-hour urinary volume of pre- and post-weight reduction were significant: *$p < 0.05$; **$p < 0.01$.

(c) Load on renal system. Dehydration will cause decreases of renal blood flow, glomerular filtration rate, and changes in urinary electrolyte concentrations (table XXIII).

(d) Losses of body proteins and minerals (fig. 9).

(e) An impairement of the thermoregulatory process.

(f) Depletion of muscle and liver glycogen stores.

(g) Influences on physical performance.

(i) A reduction in endurance induced by dehydration has been generally accepted. (ii) Whether a rapid weight loss will reduce muscular strength is debatable. (iii) Effects on maximal oxygen uptake and oxygen debt depend on the percentages of the initial weight and the duration of the weight loss period.

However, athletes who undergo weight loss are in a state of stress. Most of them show signs of dehydration as dry mouth, dizziness, drowsiness, faintness, restlessness, depressiveness or irritability, etc., and muscle cramps and weakness developed in part of the athletes.

Table XXII. (cont.)

P, beats/min			Pulse pressure, mm/Hg		
pre-WR	WR	post-WR	pre-WR	WR	post-WR
	70 ± 4.3			40 ± 0.9	
70 ± 10.7		77 ± 8.9	40 ± 10.3		$32 \pm 5.9^{1.2}$

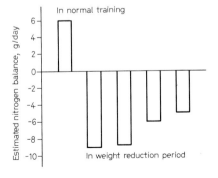

Fig. 9. Nitrogen balance of lifters in normal training and in the weight reduction period.

(2) Medical problems of long-term weight control:

Whether it is necessary for girl gymnasts to maintain long-term weight control is still a controversy and there have been different opinions, and the most important problem athletes face is 'What is the optimal weight to maintain?' Recommendations of the best body weight for this group of athletes are: the weight at which athletes achieve excellent performance in competition, get their maximal strength, speed, endurance, and the minimum percentages of body fat to permit health and effective performance.

A 3-year systematic study on a group of girl gymnasts on long-term weight control showed detrimental effects as follows [17]: (a) growth retardation; (b) menstrual disturbances; (c) malnutrition; (d) mental stress and pressure; (e) constipation; (f) muscular weakness and impairment of performance.

(3) Suggestions of nutritional improvement for athletic weight reduction:

The desire of the intense, highly competitive athlete to change weight without medical guidance usually results in hazards and abuse of medicine that may often impair health and performance. The necessity of developing safe and effective programs for weight reduction continues to be a matter of concern. The recommended method to lose excess body weight for athletic competition involves a balanced lower calorie diet and exercise. It has been accepted that the athletes will compete well if they achieve their competing weight while being well nourished, well hydrated and possessing a healthy minimum of energy reserves in the form of body fat.

As to the optimum competing weight and body fat, the AMA Committee on medical aspects has established that 7–10% of body fat is desirable in wrestlers [18]. The American College of Sports Medicine suggested that the lowest possible body weight includes at least 5% body fat, athletes with a body fat content of less than 5% of their certified weight should receive medical clearance before competition [19]. Preventive measurements emphasize that the daily caloric requirement of wrestlers should be obtained from a balanced diet; the minimal caloric intake ranges from 1,200 to 2,400 kcal/day; discourage the practice of fluid deprivation and dehydration. Forbid to use diuretics since all the diuretics will be included in the doping list.

For the purpose of preventing medical complications of reducing body weight, the intensified food and slow released multi-mineral tablet were designed. The intensified food provided 450 kcal/100 g and contains high quality protein, adequate amounts of carbohydrate and vitamins. The slow released multi-mineral tablet was designed on the basis of experimental data

Table XXIV. Hemoglobin concentrations of athlethes

Group	Hb concentration, g%	
	before WR	after WR
Supplemented	15.1 ± 1.5	15.4 ± 1.1
Nonsupplemented	14.7 ± 1.2	16.1 ± 1.5*

*$p < 0.05$.

Table XXV. Fasting blood glucose levels of athletes

Group	n	Blood glucose levels, mg%		Number of cases of hypo-glycemia
		before weight reduction	after weight reduction	
Supplemented	15	137 ± 4.2	128 ± 15.6	0
Nonsupplemented	12	101 ± 13.4	104 ± 20.6	2

Table XXVI. Incidence of ketonuria in athletes during the weight reduction period

Group	n	Incidence of ketonuria (n)
Supplemented	15	0
Nonsupplemented	12	5

and used as supplements under medical supervision [20]. The effects were as follows: (a) Body weight of athletes supplementing intensified food could be reduced, but the reducing speed was slightly slower. (b) Dehydration conditions were reduced and hemoconcentration did not seem to occur (table XXIV). (c) Hypoglycemia and ketonuria were prevented (tables XXV, XXVI). (d) The load on the cardiovascular system was decreased. (e) The intensified food replaced the body with proteins, minerals and vitamins; thus, the negative nitrogen balance, and mineral and vitamin insufficiency were corrected (fig. 10). In addition, the athletes' physical strength was improved, and the incidence of muscle cramps was reduced.

For gymnasts, etc., we suggest that weight control or reduction procedure is not needed if the athletes train normally and the body fat does not increase. Education for coaches and athletes on the physiological conse-

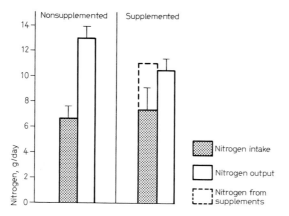

Fig. 10. Nitrogen balance of lifters with and without food supplements in the weight reduction period.

quences and medical complications which can occur as a result of long-term food restriction are important. We emphasize the necessity of assessing body compositions of athletes, discourage the athletes with body fat under 10% to take weight reduction procedures, and prohibit the single or combined use of rubber or plastic suits, steam rooms, hot boxes, sunas, laxatives, and diuretics to 'make weight'.

Nutrition improvements include increasing the energy intake to $\geq 90\%$ of the requirement and providing protein intake to 1.9 g/kg. We stress on a balanced diet and especially on the intake of foods as vegetables, fruits and milk products to assure plenty of nutrition of minerals and vitamins.

A 3-year follow-up study showed the effects as follows: (a) Comprehensive nutrition improvements made the growth rate of gymnasts greater than that of the same-aged students. (b) The nutrition status was improved and malnutrition was corrected. (c) Rational nutrition improvement did not cause body fat increase if athletes were in normal training, but lean body mass and the index of 'Ht (cm)–Weight (kg)' increased significantly.

Results of the study also suggest that comprehensive and systematic body composition investigations are valuable indices not only for evaluating training effects, but also for predicting performance capacity and guidance for body weight control of gymnasts.

However, a rational weight control method is still needed to be researched.

References

1   Chen JD, Liao GZ, Yu CY: The study of energy expenditure rate of gymnastic sports. Chin J Prevent Med 1964; 9:227–231.

2   Chen JD, Liao GZ, Yu CY: Investigation of the energy expenditure in athletes. J Beijing Med Coll 1965; 3:204–209.

3   Liao GZ, Yu CY: The study of energy expenditure rate of weight lifting. Chin J Prevent Med 1965; 10:351–353.

4   Health Institute of the Chinese Academy of Medical Sciences: Food Composition Table, ed 2, pp 368, Beijing, People's Health Publishing House, 1976.

5   Chen JD, Bai RY, Zhang BH, et al: Study of energy expenditure in Ballet Dancers. Acta Nut Sin 1986; 8:267–272.

6   Chen JD, Chen ZM, Yang ZY, et al: Research of the protein metabolism and requirements of athletes. Sports Sci 1982; 2:49–57.

7   Chen JD: Primary research of water and mineral metabolism of long distance runners. J Beijing Med Coll 1962; 1–72.

8   Chen JD, Liao GZ, Yu CY: The vitamin C metabolism of organism in sports. J Beijing Med Coll 1965; 4:282–287.

9   Chen JD, Yu XX, Nie FE: The study of vitamin C status and requirement of the gymnasts and middle-long distance runners. Chin Med J 1962; 7:454–457.

10   Chen JD, Liao GZ, Yu CY: Primary approach of the vitamin C requirement of athletes during competition period from the excretion of urinary vitamin C. Chin Med J 1963; 49:256–260.

11   Chen JD, Chen ZM, Huang GJ: The study of urinary catecholamine and blood lactic acid in functional evaluation of athletes. Sports Sci 1982; 3: 56–66.

12   Chen JD, Chen ZM, Zhang MR, et al: A study of serum protein components in evaluating the functional state of athletes. Collection of Papers on Functional Evaluation of Athletes in 1985. Changsha, 1985, pp 42–47.

13   Chen JD, Chen ZM, Zhang MR, et al: The effect of physical exercise on serum immunoglobin of human body. Chin J Sports Med 1983; 3:19–23.

14   Chen JD, Chen ZM: The relationship between the phagocytic activity of white blood cells and the blood vitamin C content of athletes. J Beijing Med Coll 1975; 1: 57–58.

15   Chen, JD, Jiao Y, Zhang MR, et al: The investigation of anemia in children and adolescent amateur athletes. J Beijing Med Coll 1978; 2: 198–201.

16   Chen JD, Yang ZY, Wu YZ, et al: Medical problems of weight lifters during the period of body weight reduction. Chin J Sports Med 1982; 1:25–29.

17   Chen JD, Yang ZY, Jiao Y, et al: Study on the nutrition and body composition of girl gymnasts during weight control. Sports Sci 1987; 7:22–25.

18   American College of Sports Medicine: Position stand on weight loss in wrestler. Med Sci Sport Exer 1980; 12:108–112.

19   Committee on Medical Aspects of Sports: Wrestling and weight control JAMA 1967; 201:541–543.

20   Chen JD, Yang ZY, Wu YZ: Study on the effects of supplementation intensified foods to lifters during weight reduction period. Acta Nutr Sin 1984; 6:97–106.

Ji Di Chen, MD, Research Division of Sports Nutrition and Biochemistry, Institute of Sports Medicine, Beijing Medical University, Beijing 100083 (China)

Subject Index

Abduction, reconstructed thumb 62
Achilles tendon
   enthesiopathy, rabbits, experimental study
     13–17
   insertion, buffer function of subtendon car-
     tilage 13
   peritendinitis, clinical investigation 7–11
Acupuncture
   effect on myofibril protein 91, 92
   effect on skeletal muscle alteration caused
     by strenuous exercise 90–93
   oblique, effect on sports injuries in skeletal
     muscles 92
Acute recurrent rhabdomyolysis, see Myoglobinuria, exercise, clinical characteristics
Aerobic training, effect on prostacyclin-
   thromboxane A_2 balance in coronary heart
     disease 81–89
Age, increase of anaerobic power 52
Aging
   dystrophic changes retarded by Tai Ji
     Quan 71
   effect on patellar tendon insertion area 12,
     13
All China Sports Federaton, nutrition 100
Anaerobic
   performance
   see also Mean power, Peak power
     trained versus untrained boys and girls,
     52–60
   power, increase with age 52

Anemia
   incidence in athletes 105, 106
   sports, relation to nutrition 105
Anoxia, stimulates release of thromboxane
   A_2 86
Anqiao 1
Apophysitis 7
Atherosclerosis, prostaglandin I_2-thrombox-
   ane A_2 imbalance 84, 86
Athletes
   abnormal electrocardiograms 34–42
   balanced diet 112
   calcium requirement 98
   copper levels 100
   ECG abnormalities 34–42
   ECG changes 36
   energy expenditure by sport 95, 96
   energy requirements 94
   enthesiopathy, clinical and pathological
     studies 7–18
   hemoglobin concentrations 111
   incidence of anemia 105, 106
   incidence of ketonuria 111
   indices for functional evaluation 102–104
   iron requirement 98
   kidney, see Hematuria
   mineral content of sweat 97
   nutritional requirements 94–101
   potassium requirement 98
   protein metabolism 94, 95
   protein requirements 97

Athletes (cont.)
  relative metabolic rate by sport 95
  sodium chloride requirement 98
  special nutrition problems 106–112
  trace mineral requirements 100
  urinary abnormalities induced by exercise
    43–51
  urinary nitrogen output 95
  water and mineral metabolism 96
  weight control 106–110
  zinc levels 100
Athletic pseudonephritis, see Hematuria
Atrioventricular block (II, III), presence in
  athletes 35–37
Badminton, players, incidence of proteinuria
  44
Ban Dang Jin exercise 3
Ban Duan Jin 1
  see also Daoyin
Basketball, players, incidence of proteinuria
  44
Beijing International Conference of Sports
  Medicine (1985) 6
Beijing Research Institute of Sports Medi-
  cine 4
Bicycling, incidence of proteinuria 44
Blood
  glucose levels, fasting, athletes 111
  lipid levels, effect of Tai Ji Quan 74, 75
  pressure
    effect of weight reduction 108
    effects of Tai Ji Quan 73
Body fat, optimum for competing 110
Body weight, optimum for competing 110
Bones, effect of Tai Ji Quan 71, 72

Calcium, daily requirement for athletes 98
Cardiac function, effects of Tai Ji Quan 73
Cardiovascular
  regulation, autonomic nervous system, ef-
    fects of Tai Ji Quan 73
  system
    effects of Tai Ji Quan 73, 74
    relationship of urinary catecholamine
      102
Cartilage
  articular

    changes during joint movement 21, 22
    normal structure 19–21
    nutrition 21
    wear and tear, influence on sports train-
      ing 26, 27
  defect, subchondral bone 29
  degenerative effects of joint immobiliza-
    tion 22
  injury
    cotton splint 32f
    pathophysiology 19–33
    pros and cons of immobilization treat-
      ment 24–26
    rehabilitation 19–33
  repair
    histochemical examination 28–31
    histological examination 28–31
    process 27–31
Casts, urinary, types 49
Catecholamine
  urinary excretion, athletes 102
  urinary, index for functional evaluation of
    athletes 102
Cathepsin D, role in cartilage 20
China, history of sports medicine 1–6
Chinese Association of Sports Medicine 4
Chinese Journal of Sports Medicine 4
Chondrocytes 19
  function 20
  lacunae buffer, function during traction 11
Chondromalacia
  incidence in athletes 26
  patellar 19
Collagen 19
  synthesis by chondrocytes 20
  wavy, function during traction 11
Copper, levels in athletes 100
Coronary heart disease
  effect of aerobic training and Qigong
    81–89
  relationship of prostaglandin I_2-thrombox-
    ane A_2 balance 84–86
Cotton splints
  advantages 26
  cartilage injury 32
  joint immobilization 25, 26
Cylindruria, exercise 49

Daoyin
characteristics 1
painting 2

Electrocardiograms, abnormal in athletes
34–42
Electroencephalogram, Tai Ji Quan exercisers
versus nonexercisers 78
Energy consumption, Tai Ji Quan exercise
76–78
Energy expenditure, sport 95, 96
Enthesiopathy
aging 12, 13
clinical and pathological studies in athletes
7–18
pathogenesis 13–16
prevention, athletes 16, 17
treatment 16, 17
Epiphysitis, animal model 14, 15
Exercise
see also Tai Ji Quan
changes in whole-blood vitamin C levels
99
effect on
hemoglobin content 106
prostaglandin I_2-thromboxane A_2
red blood cells 106
increase of urinary protein excretion 45
strenuous
effect on skeletal muscle 90, 91
skeletal muscle alteration and effect of
acupuncture 90–93
urinary abnormalities 43–51
vitamin C requirement 98, 99
Females, anaerobic performance 54–56
Femoral trochlea 19
Football hematuria, see Hematuria

Glucosaminoglycans
function 20
function during traction 11
Glucose, blood, effect of weight reduction
108
Gymnastics, incidence of proteinuria 44

Hamstring tendon 7
Hand, strength, injured versus uninjured 67

Heart, abnormalities in athletes, ECG-re-
vealed 34–42
Hematuria
diagnosis in athletes 46
exercise (10000 m), causes 46, 47
Hemoarthrosis, treatment 27
Hemoglobin
concentrations in athletes 111
effect of intensive exercise 106
effect of weight reduction 108
Hemoglobinuria, exertional 47, 48
clinical characteristics 47, 48
effect of resilient soles on athletic shoes 48
symptoms like acute intravascular hemolysis 48
Hydrocortisone injection, subtendon chondral pad 10
Hypertension, preventative effects of Tai Ji
Quan 74

Idiopathic myoglobinuria, see Myoglobinuria, exercise, clinical characteristics
Idiopathic rhabdomyolysis, see Myoglobinuria, exercise, clinical characteristics
Immobilization
joint, effects 22
pros and cons for treatment of cartilege injury 24–26
Immunity function, effect of Tai Ji Quan 76
Immunoglobulin
index for functional evaluation of athletes
102
serum, levels in athletes according to condition 104
Intraarticular hemorrhage, treatment 27
Iron, daily requirement for athletes 98

Joint
see also Cartilage, articular; Cartilage injury
articular surfaces, significance of contact
area for rehabilitation 52
capsule, role 21
effects of immobilization 22
effects of Tai Ji Quan 71, 72
effusion, treatment 27
lack of irritation on articular surface and

Joint (cont.)
    cartilage
        damage 22, 24
    movement
        changes in articular cartilage 21, 22
        lack, physiological effects 22
    surface, structure 19, 20
Jumpers' knee 7
Junctional escape, presence in athletes 40
Junctional rhythm, presence in athletes 40

Ketonuria, incidence in athletes 111

Lactic acid, blood, index for functional evalu-
    ation of athletes 102, 103
Lacunae buffer, chondrocytes, function dur-
    ing traction 11
Left anterior hemiblock, presence in athletes
    40
Left artrial rhythm, presence in athletes 40
Ligament
    insertion
        bending insertion type 8, 9
        function 11, 12
        injuries 7–18
        normal structure 7–11
        traction type 11
        trochlear type 8
        types 8–11
    reconstruction, rehabilitative protocol 25
Longevity exercise, see Daoyin
Lysosomes, role in cartilage 20

Males, anaerobic performance 54–56
Marathon running, incidence of proteinuria
    44
Matrix, cartilage, function 19, 20
Mean power
    males versus females 54–56
    trained versus untrained boys and girls
        57
Mineral metabolism, athletes 96
Muscle injuries, effect of oblique acupuncture
    in treatment 92
Myofibril, effect of acupuncture 91, 92
Myoglobinuria, exercise, clinical characteris-
    tics 49

Nitrogen balance, athletes 112
Nutrition
    relation to sports anemia 105
    requirements for athletes 94–101
    special problems in athletes 106–110
    sports, research in China 94–113

Opposition, reconstructed thumb 62
Osgood-Schlatter disease 15

Paroxysmal tachycardia, presence in athletes
    39
Patella, effects of permanent dislocation, rab-
    bits 22–24
Patella, rabbit, normal articular cartilage 20
Patellar
    dislocation, cartilage defect 30, 31
    tendon, peritendinitis
        clinical investigation 7–11
        clinical pathology 12
    tendon insertion area, effect of aging
        12–13
Peak power
    males versus females 54–56
    trained versus untrained boys and girls 57
Peritendinitis
    Achilles tendon, clinical investigation
        7–11
    patellar tendon, clinical investigation, pa-
        thology 7–12
Potassium, daily requirement for athletes 98
Premature beat, presence in athletes 39
Prostacyclin (PGI$_2$) measurement 82
Protein
    metabolism, athletes 94, 95
    requirement, athletes 97
Proteinuria, incidence according to sport, ex-
    ercise 44, 45
Proteoglycan 20

Qigong 87
    effect on synthesis of PGI$_2$ 87
    effects on prostacyclin-thromboxane A$_2$
        balance in coronary heart disease 81–89

Range of motion
    exercises for, reconstructed thumb, 64, 65

measurement, reconstructed thumb 62
thumb, uninjured versus injured 67
Red blood cells, filter rate and osmotic fragility before and after exercise 106
Relative metabolic rate, sport 95
Respiratory function, effects of Tai Ji Quan 74
Right atrial rhythm, presence in athletes 40
Right bundle branch block, incomplete, presence in athletes 37
Rotator cuff injury 7
Running, incidence of proteinuria 44

Sediments, urinary, types 49
Septic arthritis 27
Serum
    endocrine levels, effect of Tai Ji Quan 75, 76
    protein
        index for functional evaluation of athletes 102
        levels in athletes according to condition 103
'Shen' deficiency, effect of Tai Ji Quan 76
Shooting, incidence of proteinuria 44
Skating
    long-distance, incidence of proteinuria 44
    speed, incidence of proteinuria 44
Skeletal muscle
    changes after strenuous exercise, 90, 91
    effect of acupuncture after strenuous exercise-induced changes 90–93
Soccer, players, incidence of proteinuria 44
Sodium chloride, daily requirement for athletes 98
Spine flexibility, effect of Tai Ji Quan 72
Sports
    anemia, relation to nutrition 105
    cardiology 34–42
    medicine, China
        divisions 4, 5
        publications 5
        research network 5
        scientific symposiums 5
Squat jump syndrome 49
State Research Institute of Sports Science of Beijing 4

Stress, result of rapid weight loss in athletes 109, 110
Stress hematuria, see Hematuria
Subtendinous chondral pad, patellar insertion area 8
Subtendon chondral pad 9
    hyalinized and degenerated 10
    hydrocortisone injection 10
Supraventricular tachycardia, presence in athletes 39
Swimming, incidence of proteinuria 44
Synovial fluid, joint, role 21

Tachycardia, paroxysmal, presence in athletes 39
Tai Ji Quan
    anthropometric studies 70, 71
    chronic effects 70–76
    description 70
    immediate physiological changes 76–78
    physiological studies in China 70–80
Tendon
    chondrofication 16
    injuries 7–18
    insertion
        aging influence 12
        bending traction type 8, 9
        chondrofication 15
        function 11, 12
        infrapatellar, rabbit 9
        normal, rabbit 8
        pathology 12
        traction type 11
        trochlear type 8
        types 8–11
    normal structure 7–11
Tennis elbow 7
Thromboxane A_2, measurement 82
Thumb, range of motion, uninjured versus injured 67
Thumb reconstruction
    abduction 62
    functional training 61–70
    muscle strength 62
    opposition 62
    range of motion measurement 62
Trace elements, requirements for athletes 100

Training
    functional, reconstructed thumb, methods
        63–65
    intensity, urinary abnormalities 43
Transplantation, functional training, second
    toe for thumb reconstruction 61–70
T wave changes, presence in athletes 38, 39

Urinary abnormalities, *see also* Cylindruria,
    exercise; Hematuria; Hemoglobinuria exer-
    tional; Myoglobinuria, exercise; clinical
    characteristics; Proteinuria, incidence ac-
    cording to sport, exercise
    according to sport 43
    factors responsible 43, 44
    induced by exercise in athletes 43–51
    influence of attitude and temperature 43
Urinary nitrogen output 95, 97
Urinary protein excretion
    according to age 45
    increased by physical exercise 45

Ventricular rhythm, presence in athletes 40
Ventricular tachycardia, presence in athletes
    39
Vitamin C
    blood content and condition of athlete 103
    blood distribution by sport 101
    changes in whole-blood levels after exer-
        cise 99

relationship to phagocytic activity of white
    blood cells 104
requirement during exercise 98, 99
Vitamins, daily requirements for athletes 100

Water metabolism, athletes 96
Weight
    control
        long-term, effects 110
        problems in athletes 106–110
    reduction
        effect on blood glucose levels 108
        effect on blood pressure 108
        effect on hemoglobin levels 108
        rapid, health problems 108–110
    lifting, incidence of proteinuria 44
White blood cells, relationship between pha-
    gocytic activity and vitamin C content 104
Wingate Anaerobic Test 54
Wolff-Parkinson-White syndrome, presence
    in athletes 39
Wu Quin Xi, 1
    see also Daoyin

Xing Qi, *see* Daoyin

Yi Jin Jing 1
    see also Daoyin

Zinc, levels in athletes 100